MEDICAL RESEARCH DESIGN AND DATA ANALYSIS

Xu-Feng Huang, MD, PhD, DSc
Distinguished Professor of Medical Science

Illawarra Health and Medical Research Institute
School of Medical, Indigenous, and Health Sciences
The University of Wollongong
Australia
2022

Ashahi-Maple

National Library of Australia Cataloguing-in-Publication Data is available.

First published in Australia in 2022
by Ashahi-Maple©, Inc.

ISBN 978-0-6454760-0-2

TO OUR FAMILIES

Preface

Who is this book for? Today, clinicians, health workers, and medical researchers require comprehensive knowledge to read literature, design research projects, and analyze data. This textbook provides the theoretical background and practical skills needed to read, interpret, appraise, and write research papers. Information is presented straightforwardly and placed into the context of actual research studies, helping the reader make real-life connections.

The aim of this book is to: (1) develop the ability to read, understand, and evaluate current professional literature, (2) learn research methods and data analysis, (3) gain the skills and knowledge required to undertake and interpret research, and (4) have the skills to critically appraise a research paper in the medical, biomedical and health science fields.

Research design. A strategy addresses the research question by using appropriate methods and techniques. The research question will determine the research design and measurements. Here, we introduce the nature of research; evidence-based medicine; research design basics; descriptive, observational, and correlation studies; randomized controlled trials; sample size determination; and research validity, bias, and confounders.

Data analysis. A process of data generates meaningful insight and supports decision-making. Starting with the basics, we describe the data type and distribution, introduce how to measure the data and variables, construct valid hypotheses, and then depict statistical methods, including parametric and nonparametric analysis. These skills will help you collect, sort, condense, model, and evaluate the research data, which are the foundations for outcome presentation, discussion, and conclusion.

Project appraisal. A project requires a compelling story in a defined structure, communicating the science to the reader. Correct research design and analysis lead to high-quality outcomes and avoid misinterpretations.

Dr. Xu-Feng Huang, MD, PhD, DSc

Contents

PART ONE

Research Design

The research design must focus on the research question of the project. Therefore, it is essential to evaluate the research potential of the question before beginning the process of designing a research project and estimating the amount of work required. Only once this is done can a research project be produced.

Keynotes for Research Project Design

Formulate a research question: It must be accurate, simple, focused, and supported by reliable information; otherwise, the project will be too broad. Therefore, a clear and precise research question is of central importance.

Assemble the best evidence: It must be comprehensive and relevant. A thorough understanding of the existing literature is essential.

Research design: To devise a research design that focuses on the question.

Select the type of data to be collected: Different questions will require different data. For example, it could be continuous data or categorical data.

Anticipate the outcome: When designing the study, it is necessary to have clear expectations before performing the research.

Some key questions in evaluating the research design:

- Has the work been done before?
- Does it fill a gap in the current research?
- Is it innovative or incremental?
- How do you find the best evidence to justify the study?

CHAPTER 1

Introduction

TOPIC OUTLINE

- Types of research questions
- Correlational research
- Cause and effect research
- Primary research
- Research location
- Descriptive statistics
- Inferential statistics

What Is Research?

Research is to gather information, make judgments on existing data, and develop new knowledge and skills to address scientific questions. It is a systematic process of augmenting existing knowledge and generating new knowledge.

Medical research aims to address health and medical or clinical questions. Research objects can be human subjects, experimental animals, and cells.

Human Research

Survey study: The researcher asks participants about their knowledge, experience, attitudes, and preferences. This can be a list of questions specifically formulated to elicit information from a sample size of subjects through their answers and responses. A survey study could be conducted via phone, mail, or street desk. The outcome focuses on drawing meaningful conclusions instead of quantitative work.

Observational study: An *observational study* draws inferences from a population sample. The independent variable is not changed or manipulated. There are three primary observational studies: cross-sectional (or prevalence study), case-control, and cohort. These studies are helpful when ethical or practical problems preclude performing a randomized controlled trial. For example, a high-fat diet is a risk factor for cardiovascular disease, and assigning subjects to a high-fat diet is unethical.

Experimental study: An *experimental study* belongs to an interventional study. Researchers have direct control of the conditions under which it occurs. As a result, the investigation can offer the most substantial evidence about a possible cause-and-effect relationship. *Randomized controlled trials,* for example, are a leading form of human experimental study.

Types of Research Questions

Basic Research Question

A *basic research question* typically deals with theoretical concepts and has no immediate concern with application or external validity. Instead, the scientist's curiosity or interest usually drives it. Aiming to expand human knowledge, it has no apparent commercial value.

Examples of basic research questions are as follows:

- How does the liver metabolize glucose?
- What are the genetic codes for the human brain?
- What is the role of neurotrophic factors in metabolic syndrome?

Applied Research Question

The *applied research question* is undertaken with a specific question or application for the general public. It aims to solve practical problems.

Examples of applied research questions are as follows:

- Everyday problem: Will more dietary fiber intake improve health? Does fish oil intake reduce the incidence of diet-induced obesity?
- Illness or disease cure: Can dietary fiber be used to improve gut health?
- Innovative technology: Can we improve the resolution of a magnetic resonance imaging machine to find a tumor in the body in its early stage?

Clinical Research Question

The question involves specific patients through interventions, prognostic factors, and risk exposure.

A clinical research question may do the following:

Address pathological conditions: For example, using tissue samples from patients in research.

Investigate the function of a specific organ: For example, the heart, kidney, or gut.

Monitor behavioral changes: For example, learning, memory, and cognitive function. Usually, a clinical research question does not address the mechanism or involve the general public.

Examples of clinical research questions:

- Does pain medication administration at the surgical incision time last twenty-four hours after surgery?

- Do people diagnosed with dementia experience depression?
- How can cachexia be prevented in cancer patients receiving radiation and chemotherapy?

Correlational Research

Correlational research aims to answer two variables that may or may not correlate. It is non-experimental research. For example, what is the relationship between A and B or A, B, and C? Correlational research does not address causal and consequence effects.

Examples:

- Listening to music lowers blood pressure. A researcher hypothesizes that listening to music lowers blood pressure. A study can collect data on participants' listening to music duration and blood pressure, followed by association analysis.
- Is there a relationship between intelligence quotient (IQ) and self-esteem?
- It was hypothesized that the longer couples stay together, the more aligned they are in their opinions.

Cause-and-Effect Research

Cause-and-effect research belongs to an experimental study. It aims to establish a cause-and-effect relationship.

Examples:

- It was hypothesized that the fish oil capsule reduces bad cholesterol if patients take it regularly.

- Regular exercise improves cognitive function in dementia patients.
- Metformin suppresses food intake in overweight people.

Primary and Secondary Research

Primary research requires a researcher to collect or generate new data instead of relying on data collected from previous studies. The researcher is directly involved in the data collection.

Secondary research is also called *desk research*. It relies on harvesting existing data from the literature. The researcher collects and summarizes the data for overall effects or outcomes. The procedure of secondary research involves the collection, evaluation, analysis, synthesis, and summary of existing research.

Research Location

Laboratory research: The study is conducted under controlled conditions permitting tighter control over the experiment.

Field research: The study is conducted in a natural environment to observe the subjects in their setting.

Table 1 Features of qualitative and quantitative research

Qualitative research	Quantitative research
Research strategies that emphasize words rather than numbers in data collection and analysis	Research strategies that emphasize numbers in data collection and analysis
Qualitative research is focused on generating theories (captures and uses lived experiences in the social world and the meanings that individuals give to these experiences from their own perspective).	Quantitative research is focused on testing theories
Understands meaning, belief, attribute, and subjective experience	Studies differences and association and establishes cause-and-effect relationships

The aim of the research always determines the type of study to be used. The research methods and designs should directly address the research question.

Descriptive Statistics

Descriptive statistics measure a group's characteristics without generalizing those statistics beyond that group. Therefore, it is about sample statistics. For example, the sample mean (M) and standard deviation (SD).

Features of descriptive data or summary analyses: The aim is to describe or summarize the data, which is the information collected from experiments, surveys, or historical records. It can be either quantitative or qualitative research.

Descriptive statistics measure central tendency (i.e., mean, median, mode, range) and variations (e.g., standard deviation).

Example of descriptive statistics:

- Range, including maximum and minimum values
- Mean, median, and mode
- Sample size
- Measurement of data variation

Descriptives

	Disease			Statistic	Std. Error
BMI	Bipolar	Mean		29.53	.550
		95% Confidence Interval for Mean	Lower Bound	28.39	
			Upper Bound	30.66	
		5% Trimmed Mean		29.39	
		Median		28.73	
		Variance		7.551	
		Std. Deviation		2.748	
		Minimum		26	
		Maximum		36	
		Range		11	
		Interquartile Range		3	
		Skewness		.676	.464
		Kurtosis		.245	.902

The table shows descriptive statistics generated by SPSS computer analysis software. The analysis includes twenty-five patients who have bipolar disorders. The report shows the body mass index (BMI) data (BMI = weight in kg/height in m^2). Here, the BMI mean and standard deviation are 29.53 ± 2.75. The lower and upper bounds give the lower end and upper end of the 95% confidence interval (CI) of the mean (95% CI, 28.39, 30.66).

BMI range was 11, from 26 to 36. Skewness was 0.676, moderately skewed. A normality test should be performed in this case because the skewness is not in the normal range. Given the small sample size, the Shapiro-Wilk Test should be used for the normality test. Here, kurtosis is within a normal range, 0.25.

Inferential Statistics

Inferential statistics aims to generalize unknown population parameters based on a representative sample. For example, you test a drug in a small group seeking to predict if the drug could work for a population. Therefore, the collected sample needs to represent the population accurately.

Estimation: Inferential statistics can use sample statistics to estimate population parameters. The samples can be either a single value or a range of values, for example, using the sample mean 36.5^{0}C body temperature as a point to estimate a population mean body temperature. Or use the sample mean height range (1.6 meters to 1.8 meters) to estimate a population mean height.

Hypothesis testing: Researchers formulate a hypothesis about the population and then collect the sample data referring to the hypothesis. For example, researchers want to test the idea that dietary fiber reduces cholesterol in a population, using baseline and after-intervention means calculated from a sample.

It is noted that inferential statistics can be used to make suggestions but cannot be used to prove or conclude causal or consequence relationships definitively.

Software used for data analysis: Computer software is used in medical data analysis. The common ones are (1) SPSS, Statistical

Package for the Social Sciences, 2) SAS, Statistical Analysis System, and (3) STAT, a statistical software package (meta-analysis).

ASK YOURSELF

- What are the main types of human studies?
- What are the main types of research questions?
- What are the definitions of observational and experimental research?
- What are the differences between an association hypothesis and a causal hypothesis?
- What are the differences between descriptive and inferential statistics?
- What are the differences between primary and secondary research?

CHAPTER 2

Evidence-Based Medicine

TOPIC OUTLINE

- Criteria
- Assessing the problem
- Acquiring the evidence
- Appraising the evidence
- Applying the evidence
- Evaluating performance

Evidence-based medicine (EBM) is a systematic approach to a clinical problem that integrates the best research evidence with clinical expertise and patient values. "A twenty-first-century clinician who cannot critically read a study must be as unprepared as one who cannot take blood pressure or examine the cardiovascular system" (Sackett et al., 1996).

In evaluating the evidence, you must consider its origin, validity, and value to patients. Then, gather the information that will help to contextualize the results and apply them to practice.

Criteria

What are the three essential criteria of evidence-based medicine?

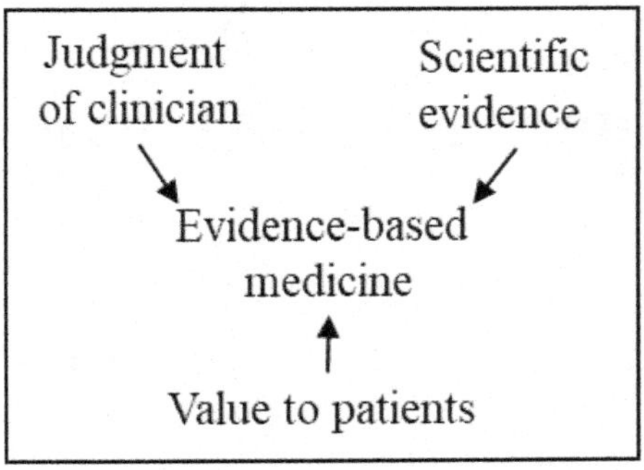

A flowchart shows that the three essential components are integrated into evidence-based medicine. They are the clinician's or expert's judgment, solid scientific evidence, and value or benefits to patients.

Non-Evidence-Based Medicine

Evidence based on clinical experience alone without conducting any form of scientific experimentation or intervention is not evidence-based medicine.

The following examples are *not* evidence-based medicine.

- Basing their conclusions exclusively on their clinical experience, a doctor claims that the only appropriate treatment for headaches is sleep.
- A doctor applying a primary mechanism or pathophysiological principle to clinical practice, for example, using melatonin to reduce inflammatory cytokine production after reading in a research journal that it worked in a study that tested it on inflammatory brain cells in a cell culture.
- A doctor relies on common sense or opinions for new treatments or clinical decisions.

- A doctor generates practical guidelines for practice based on clinical experience.

Five-step process of evidence-based medicine

Assessing the Problem

Researchers need to translate a clinical problem into a *testable* or *answerable* question. Unfortunately, there can be many unstructured clinical or practical questions. These questions can be vague or complex, hard to answer, or not answerable.

Researchers need to convert these unstructured questions into answerable questions or testable hypotheses. An appropriate question should have clearly defined (1) patient problem, (2) intervention, (3) comparison, and (4) outcome, which is a structured PICO format (Akobeng, 2005).

For example, obesity is a risk factor, especially when there is an elevated low-density lipoprotein level (LDL, > 5.5 mmol/l). LDL is "bad" cholesterol because it collects in the walls of the blood vessels. So researchers want to use dietary fiber supplements to reduce high LDL in obese subjects. The question will be: Does dietary fiber supplementation reduce high LDL compared with no dietary fiber in obese subjects with high LDL? Or, we hypothesize that dietary fiber supplementation normalizes high LDL levels in obese subjects. Here, the problem is high LDL in obese patients. The intervention is dietary fiber, the comparison is no dietary fiber, and the outcome is LDL levels, a structured PICO format.

Acquire the Evidence

You should search the evidence available in the literature after the clinical or practical problem is converted to a testable question.

The first step is to define the keywords for searching the literature. You should use the keywords in the question that you have raised. For example, from the question mentioned above, the keywords for the search are "obesity" (problem), "dietary fiber" (intervention), and "LDL levels" (outcomes).

The next step is to choose the database. Many online medical databases are available, including PubMed, Medline, Google Scholar, Web of Science, Cochrane Library, and EMBASE. PubMed and Medline are widely used databases for searching biomedical literature, which is very useful for fundamental research. Cochrane database collects many systematic reviews and other secondary analytical research and clinical trials that are very helpful for clinical research.

The searching strategy can use the keywords "and" and "or" combinations. You may use two or three keywords simultaneously. I would recommend using two keywords search first, as it is simple. Sometimes, you find too many articles under one topic. In this case, you can use limitations, such as publication type, years, or human only.

Appraising the Evidence

There are many criteria that you can use to appraise a research paper. The decision of what criteria to use depends on the purpose of your investigation. Doing clinical research will be different from basic or mechanistic research. For example, a clinical researcher may consider the feasibility and benefits to the patients. However, a mechanistic study may emphasize cause, precision, and effect size.

Generally speaking, you may use some criteria to evaluate the quality of medical evidence.

Validity: Assess whether the study is valid by checking the internal and external validities. You will need to determine whether or not the outcome is by chance. Also, you need to evaluate if the result is biased.

Effect size: A larger effect size gives more confidence as a piece of evidence than a small effect size. You may examine the effect size by comparing the intervention group with the control group or pre-treatment and post-treatment groups.

Precision: The sample size should be large enough to conclude the outcomes. Conversely, a small sample size will likely lead to a false conclusion. Also, the measurements should be accurate and precise as you consider the evidence.

Patient value: The evidence is valid for clinical or practical usefulness. Having unreliable evidence applied to clinical practice could cause harm or no effects, which wastes resources.

Medical Evidence

Medical evidence is the outcome or information generated by various studies. Medicine has a long history of research on diagnosis, cause, pathology, treatment, and prevention. Multiple types of tools or methods can produce the evidence. These methods have a restricted structure to obtain standardized information or evidence. The critical point is to make sure that the evidence is accurate.

The figure shows the hierarchy of study types in terms of evidence. The types of medical evidence can be ranked from most to least significant. The higher the study type is in the hierarchy, the more substantial the evidence. Conversely, the lower the order, the weaker the evidence. A greater level of trust should be in the higher evidence study type.

Medical Evidence Levels

Medical evidence 1: Systematic review and meta-analysis are at the top of the pyramid. The evidence is from the review and meta-analysis of all papers in the field over many years. Therefore, the conclusion has a much greater value. The practice procedure should be systematically developed to enable practitioners and patients to follow it. A systematic review will summarize the evidence; eliminate bias, ambiguities, and confoundings; and make conclusions utilizing all current data. Meta-analysis uses statistics and quantitative analysis to address specific questions and draw conclusions about existing knowledge.

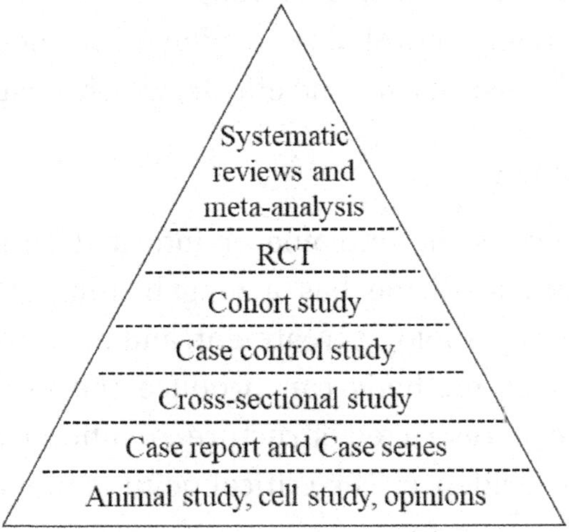

Medical evidence 2 is from a randomized controlled trial (RCT). An appropriate randomized controlled trial generates the outcomes supporting the causal and consequential relationship. Furthermore, a quasi-experimental design is used when a randomized controlled trial is unfeasible or presents ethical issues. There are many types of quasi-experimental methods. For example, a study has two groups, where one group receives the intervention and one does not, but there is no randomization of the sample allocation.

Medical evidence 3 is from a cohort study. A cohort study is a longitudinal study with two groups of participants. One group receives exposure to the risk, and one does not. Then the two groups are monitored over time to see if they develop the disease. The researcher investigates outcomes during disease development.

Medical evidence 4 is from a case-control study. Such a study starts with a disease condition followed by comparing the subjects with or without the previous exposure risks, for example, the individuals with mild cognitive deficits compared to those without cognitive deficits. Then the study investigates the variables that might result from the disease (e.g., metabolic syndrome, obesity, stressful lifestyle). The evidence generated from this study determines the differences and associations between the variables, but it does not establish a cause-and-consequence relationship.

Medical evidence 5 is from cross-sectional studies. Practically, a cross-sectional study is an observational study comparing the differences and the associations between variables. It does not address a cause-and-consequence relationship.

Medical evidence 6 is from a case series and case report. This type of study has a small number of subjects or could have one case only. It reports on unusual cases and aims to develop possible hypotheses for further investigation. It is based on expert opinion and with no appropriate research method applied.

Evidence Validity between Research Types

Because randomized trials and systematic reviews are much more likely to inform us and much less likely to mislead us, they are the "gold standard" for judging whether a treatment does more good than harm.

On the other hand, evidence-based medicine is not limited to randomized controlled trials, systematic reviews, and meta-analyses. It is essential to consider cohort, case-control, and cross-sectional studies. However, it would be best if you could avoid non-experimental approaches for strong conclusions since they frequently lead to false-positive findings.

Applying the Evidence

After you have decided that the evidence can address the problem or question, it is time for you to consider applying the evidence to the patients. Again, the decisive factors are the expert's opinion, the patient's value, and risk. In practice, evidence should inform practice, including application design and measurements. A successful application should show if the evidence works.

Evaluating Performance

Researchers or practitioners should evaluate the performance after incorporating evidence-based medicine into their practice. They need to consider a process to find empirical evidence demonstrating the effectiveness. You then determine the relevance of that evidence to a particular practical situation. Finally, practitioners should use appropriate measurements to determine if the intervention has an intended or expected outcome.

Researchers need to formulate answerable questions, find good evidence, evaluate the evidence, and integrate clinical expertise and patient's values with the evidence leading to an acceptable management strategy (Straus and Sackett, 1998).

In the Information Era, How Can We Keep Up with New Information?

There are a lot of medical research papers out there. It is unknown how many medical articles are published annually, but we know about thirty thousand medical journals. For example, there were about seventy-five clinical trials and eleven systematic reviews a day (Bastian et al., 2010). How can you possibly keep your knowledge updated with this amount of information? Many practitioners and doctors maintain an old scope of expertise; however, keeping up with the current literature is vital. Therefore, it is crucial to devise a way to know which information is essential for your work.

Keep in mind that systematic reviews and meta-analyses are much more informative and reliable in providing solid evidence. Randomized controlled trials and experimental studies are acceptable for consideration; however, a single cross-sectional, case-control, or case report is less convincing and requires to be treated with caution. Nevertheless, the description above may help you to determine how to search for practical knowledge.

ASK YOURSELF
▪ What are the criteria for evidence-based medicine? ▪ What are the five-step processes for evidence-based medicine? ▪ What are the essential components of constructing a testable question? ▪ How many types of scientific evidence does that evidence-based medicine include? ▪ What are the critical elements to appraise medical evidence? ▪ What is your strategy for searching for a piece of medical evidence?

CHAPTER 3

Research Design

TOPIC OUTLINE

- Research design basics
- Study design in cell, animal, and clinical research
- The research design for specific questions
- Descriptive research
- Observational and correlational research
- Randomized controlled trial

The research design is about an overall strategy for addressing the research questions. It requires *organizing* the study's components logically and coherently to address the research questions effectively.

Three essential components for a research project design:

1) To determine what type of research will be suitable to address the question.
2) To determine what will be measured and what techniques will be used.
3) To determine how to collect and analyze the data.

Research Design Basics

TOPIC OUTLINE

- Literature review
- Meta-analysis
- Data variables
- Between-subject design
- Within-subject design
- Mixed design
- Factorial design
- A 2x2 factorial design
- A 2x3 factorial design

Literature Review

A literature review is essential for a research project design. Doing a literature review helps you find relevant papers, analyze the data, understand the debates, and find research gaps requiring research. The primary goal of a literature review is to identify the research gap, justify a need for research, learn the knowledge and method under a specific topic, and provide your opinion. A literature review should contain the background, knowledge review, discussion (research gap, advance appraisal), conclusion, and recommendations.

When doing a literature review, we advise you to put more weight on systematic review and meta-analysis than any other type of study. This is because these reviews make conclusions from multiple studies and are less likely to lead to a mistake. Usually, a systematic review gathers all available primary research using clearly defined, systematic methods to answer a specific question.

Meta-analysis belongs to the data analysis using statistical methods to calculate an overall effect. The approach is to use the data from published primary studies with the same research question. It aims to generate a quantitative summary of the overall impact on a specified topic. Therefore, a meta-analysis is a statistical process of analyzing and combining results from several similar studies.

The literature review should include individual papers that are relevant and critical to your research topic. However, avoid over-citing the paper unnecessarily; articles of low quality can mislead your research direction.

Data Variables

The variables include independent, dependent, and control variables. Because the variables should directly relate to the research aim, choosing the correct independent variable and measuring the right dependent variable becomes critical for a good research design.

Independent variable: A manipulated variable is an independent variable, for example, male or female, a high-fat or high-fiber diet. The independent variable does not depend on that of another.

Dependent variable: A responsible variable is a dependent variable, as its value depends on the independent or manipulated variable. The dependent variable is what you measure or observe in the experiment.

Control variable: A control variable is a non-manipulated variable, e.g., the whole experiment was performed in the dark. A controlled variable is a variable that remains unchanged. The researcher can measure it but does not manipulate it; e.g., a dim light, 0.25 lux, was used in a rat study.

Examples: Independent variable versus dependent variable.

Can you distinguish the independent and dependent variables in the following questions?

- Is a good night's sleep critical to a crossword puzzle performance? In this case, the independent variable is sleep and if one has slept poorly or well. The dependent variable is one's performance, since this depends on sleep quality.
- Is gender a deciding factor in performance in math? Here, men and women are the independent variables, whereas math performance is the dependent variable.
- The lecturer asks twenty students to do a math test with a maximum score of 100. In this case, the students are the independent variable. The scores are the dependent variable, depending on individual students.

Between-Subjects Design

A *between-subjects design* compares the effects between groups where every subject receives one condition only. The between-subjects design is conceptually simple, and no time and learning effects are involved.

A between-subject *simple* design tests each participant in only one condition, e.g., with or without drug treatment. A between-subject *factorial* design manipulates the independent variables between subjects.

1. A between-subjects simple design

	Group 1	Group 2
Treatment	+	-
No treatment	-	+

Example: A between-subject simple design has one treatment and one no-treatment (control) as group 1 and group 2.

2. A between-subjects simple design

	Group 1	Group 2	Group 3
No treatment	+		
Drug A - low dose		+	
Drug A - high dose			+

Example: A between-subject simple design has one no-treatment group and low and high doses of the drug A groups; therefore, there are three groups.

3. A between-subject factorial design

	Group 1	Group 2	Group 3
No treatment	+		
Drug A		+	
Drug B			+

Example: A between-subject factorial design has one no-treatment group and drug A and B groups. Drug A and drug B are two different drugs; therefore, here is a factorial design. You can compare the effects of drug A, drug B, and no drug treatments.

A Within-Subjects Design

A *within-subjects design* is that the same subject tests under multiple conditions. The within-subjects design is more efficient in sample size and controls bias and confounding factors. This type of design tests each subject in all conditions, e.g., baseline and after treatments. A within-subject factorial design manipulates the independent variables within-subjects, e.g., young and old age, drug A and drug B, or male and female.

A within-subject simple design

	Baseline	After treatment
One group	+	+

Example: A within-subjects simple design has one group with the dependent variable(s) measured at baseline and after treatment(s).

A within-subjects factorial design

		Baseline	After treatment
Group 1	No treatment	+	+
Group 2	Drug A	+	+
Group 3	Drug B	+	+

Example: Here is one example that a within-subjects factorial design has one no-treatment group (control) and drug A and drug B treatment groups. The dependent variables can be measured at baseline and after the treatment(s).

Mixed Design

A *mixed design* combines a between-subjects design with a within-subjects design. The goal is to examine the differences between the groups and the changes within the group. Therefore, a mixed design can manipulate one independent variable between subjects and another within subjects.

Example: A researcher chooses smokers as a within-subject factor by testing the same participants both while smoking and not smoking. Also, the researcher might select satiety as a between-subjects factor by testing hungry or full. Each condition (smoking or hungry) is tested in two of the four conditions.

	Group 1	Group 2	Group 3	Group 4
Smoking	-	-	+	+
Hungry	-	+	-	+

Factorial Design

A *factorial design* aims to avoid misleading conclusions when variable interaction is present. This type of design estimates the effect of an outcome variable at several levels of the other independent variables. The design consists of two or multiple independent variables, each having two or more levels.

The factorial design can increase the external validity of the study. It allows the researcher to manipulate multiple variables simultaneously, expanding its range of applicability. For example, a study investigates exercise and nutrition on an outcome variable.

Multiple independent variables are the variables in different categories, e.g., male and female; exercise and nutrition. The research question can be how exercise and fish oil supplements affect cognition in the elderly. What is the effect of expectancy on anxiety-induced intention to smoke? The factorial design allows us to answer more complicated research questions than a single independent variable.

Interaction between the independent variables may or may not depend on each other. Researchers, for example, found an interaction between exercise and saturated fat intake because the effect of exercise depended on whether subjects were high or low saturated fat eaters; therefore, there is likely an interaction between exercise and fat intake.

Multiple levels of a single independent variable have the variables in the same category, e.g., nil, low, and high doses of the same compound; adolescence, adult, and old age of the population. For example, the research question can be "the effect of metformin lowering the blood glucose levels depends on the low or high dose." This design allows us to address more sophisticated research questions than using a single level of an independent variable.

The factorial design has multiple independent variables in an experiment. Each independent variable can have two or more levels combined with two or more levels of other independent variables. Each combination becomes an experimental group.

A 2x2 Factorial Design

A *2x2 factorial design* allows researchers to understand the effects of two independent variables on a single outcome variable. It combines two independent variables, each with two levels.

2 x 2 factorial design

		Independent variable 2	
		Level 1	**Level 2**
Independent variable 1	Level 1	One dependent variable, 4 groups	
	Level 2		

	BMI25-29	**BMI30-34**
20 min exercise/day	*body weight changes in 4 weeks*	
2 hours exercise/day	*4 groups*	

Example:

Suppose an exercise physiologist wants to understand the effects of exercise (twenty minutes versus two hours) and overweight or obesity indicated by body mass index (BMI 25–29 versus BMI 30–34) on body weight change over a four-week research program.

The above study requires a 2x2 factorial design because two independent variables have two levels for each. This design allows researchers to analyze the interaction, main effects, and mean values.

An interaction effect may occur when the exercise variable's effect (independent variable 1) on the body weight changes (dependent variable) depending on the level of the BMI (independent variable 2). The question to be addressed is, does exercise impact body weight depending on BMI? Conversely, does the effect of BMI on body weight changes depend on the exercise levels in this program?

Furthermore, you may find the main effect of exercise on body weight changes and the mean outcomes of the body weight changes after exercising for twenty minutes and two hours per day for four weeks. Also, you may find the main effect of BMI on body weight changes after this four-week research program and the mean body weight changes among BMI 25–29 and BMI 30–34 after these four-week exercises.

An analysis of a 2×2 factorial design requires two-way ANOVA to determine whether exercise and BMI interact with the dependent variable.

Here is an example of interpreting the output of a two-way ANOVA for a 2x2 factorial design. If the p-value for the interaction between exercise and BMI is > 0.05, there is no interaction effect between exercise and BMI. In this case, no further analysis will be required; however, if the p-value is < 0.05, you should perform a post hoc analysis to determine the differences between the groups. For example, if the p-value associated with exercise is < 0.05, it means that exercise significantly affects body weight changes. On the other hand, if the p-value associated with BMI is < 0.05, BMI size may affect body weight changes.

You may plot these means to visualize the effects of the independent variables on the dependent variable.

A 2x3 Factorial Design

A *2x3 factorial design* allows the researcher to investigate the effects of two independent variables on a single dependent variable. This type of design has two levels on one independent variable and three on another; therefore, there will be six experimental groups. The purpose is to analyze the main and association effects, which are explained in the example below.

2 x 3 factorial design		Independent variable 2		
		Level 1	Level 2	Level 3
Independent variable 1	Level 1	One dependent variable, 6 groups		
	Level 2			
		Adolescent	Adult	Old
	Male	e.g., the dependent variable is blood glucose levels, 6 groups		
	Female			

For example, suppose an endocrinologist wants to understand the effect of age (adolescent, adult, and old) and gender (male and female) on the blood glucose levels of a particular population. The case is an example of a 2x3 factorial design because there are two independent variables: one has two levels, and another has three. There is only one dependent variable, which is blood glucose levels. This study has six experimental groups.

Analysis of a 2x3 factorial design can perform a two-way ANOVA to test whether or not there are main effects, association effects between the independent and the dependent variables, and interaction effects.

The main effects that one independent variable has on the dependent variable can be broken down as follows:

The main effect of age on blood glucose levels:

- The mean level of blood glucose in adolescence.
- The mean level of blood glucose in adults.
- The mean level of blood glucose in the elderly.

The main effect of gender on blood glucose levels:

- The mean level of blood glucose in males.
- The mean level of blood glucose in females.

The interaction effect may occur when both age and gender affect blood glucose levels. This means that one independent variable's effect on the dependent variable depends on the level of the other independent variable.

- Does the effect of age on blood glucose levels depend on gender?
- Does the effect of gender on blood glucose levels depend on age?

Interpretation of these two-way ANOVA outcomes is as follows:

1) If the p-value associated with age is < 0.05, the age of subjects has a statistically significant effect on blood glucose levels.

2) If the p-value associated with sex is < 0.05, males or females significantly affect blood glucose levels.

3) The p-value for the interaction between age and sex is < 0.05. This means there is no interaction effect between age and sex.

ASK YOURSELF

- What are the aims of a literature review?
- What are the differences between a meta-analysis and a systematic review?
- What are the four types of research data variables?
- What is a between-subjects design?
- What is a within-subjects design?
- What is a mixed design?
- What is a factorial design?
- Can you design an example of a two-by-two factorial design?
- Can you come up with an example of a two-by-three factorial design?

Study Design in the Cell, Animal, and Clinical Research

TOPIC OUTLINE

- *In vitro* research
- *In vivo* research
- Preclinical research
- Clinical research
- Open, single-blind, and double-blind trial
- Experimental control group

In Vitro Study

In vitro study occurs in a laboratory by studying cells, tissues, or microorganisms in a testing tube or petri dish. It looks at biological processes, pathology, or drug action mechanisms. Also, it provides insights into how the cells respond to risk factors or candidate compounds in a controlled and isolated environment.

The advantage is to perform more detailed analyses and examine the effects (e.g., doses and time effects) in a large sample of in vitro rather than in vivo subjects. In addition, in vitro studies can avoid potential confounding factors that in vivo studies have. However, the disadvantage is that it cannot represent a full living situation; therefore, it is necessary to explain in vivo results cautiously.

The in vitro models include healthy, diseased, or gene-mutated models. For example, normal cells are harvested from normal tissue into a cell culture medium for testing. Cells can be from a specific organ of animals or humans for primary cell culture. Cell lines are mostly from tumor tissue or genetically engineered immortal cells. Cell lines offer low-cost platforms to study a compound's biological or pharmacological effect. Today, gene technology shows how cells respond to the compounds under specific gene manipulations. In addition, two-dimensional and three-dimensional cell cultures are used to screen possible candidate compounds for the disease, deliver the drugs, and make the medical device for diagnosis. Organ-on-a-chip is a technology that studies cells on a chip of many different types.

Notably, these technologies can help examine if novel compounds have toxic or carcinogenic effects on targeted cells. For example, the researcher collects cells from colon cancer patients, followed by screening or testing candidate compounds. Another example is in vitro fertilization technique. It treats infertility, where fertilization occurs in a laboratory using an egg from an ovary and placing it in a petri dish with donated sperm. Then, a doctor can implant the fertilized egg into the uterus for developing embryos.

In Vivo Research

In vivo research applies investigation in animal models and humans. It broadly applies to studying anatomy, physiology, pathology, pathophysiology, genetics, and various drug trials. Animal model studies are a middle ground between cell-based or in vitro and clinical trials. For example, in a candidate drug study, you may apply an animal model study to investigate the mechanism, safety, and efficacy before a clinical trial.

Most experimental animals share similarities in anatomy and physiology with humans, such as rodents, primates, dogs, and rabbits. In addition, experimental animals from the same species are genetically identical; therefore, investigators can study research questions within sophisticated organisms using a relatively small sample size compared with humans. Mice are commonly used for research because of their size, easy handling, fast reproduction, and relatively low cost. Also, mice share 95% of their genes with humans (Pennacchio, 2003). This is why it is common for researchers to use mice to examine the safety and efficacy of candidate drugs in a preclinical trial.

It is noted that in vivo study has strict regulations for performance due to ethics requirements.

Preclinical Research

Preclinical research uses experimental animals to study a drug, procedure, or treatment likely to be effective for humans. It is common to examine a candidate drug's toxicity, efficacy, and metabolism using a preclinical study before conducting human clinical trials. Before investigating a new drug in people, we must determine whether it can cause toxicity. Preclinical research can be observational, pilot, intervention, or mechanistic, with possible clinical application.

Preclinical research includes animal-based (in vivo) and cell-based (in vitro) studies or the two combined studies. The studies require good laboratory practices (GLP).

Not all in vitro or in vivo studies have to be preclinical studies. Many studies investigate the biological process, primary mechanism, or pathology, which have no intention for a clinical application.

Animal Models:

Sometimes, a researcher must use experimental animal models because of practical or ethical issues. Many experimental animals, such as mice, rats, and other species, can be used to mimic certain aspects of human physiology or disease. Many diseased animal models are beneficial in addressing the research questions, such as diet-induced, gene mutation-induced, and pharmacological-induced models. Animal models can help to generate knowledge about the basic science of disease and its prevention and treatment.

Examples:

- Researchers can inactivate a gene by replacing it or disrupt a gene with a fake piece of DNA called *knockout*, e.g., knockout mice. A gene knockout means the complete elimination or permanent alteration of the gene from an organism. Therefore, that gene loses its function.
- *Gene knockdown* reduces the expression level in an organism. For example, specific RNA interference (RNAi) can reduce that gene's expression levels. Therefore, this technique can examine the gene function without removing that gene.
- *Gene knock-in* is the opposite of gene knockout. Knock-in inserts a foreign gene into the organism's genome.

Cell-Based Models:

Cell models are cell lines, primary cultured cells, and stem cells. The research using cell models can give an insight into the mechanism of action for further intervention. Cell work has been beneficial for many drug studies. For example, virtually all anti-cancer drugs have used cell models to test their efficacy and toxicity.

Study Design of Preclinical Research:

The principle of preclinical research design is similar to human clinical studies. Preclinical research allows an investigation of the cause-and-effect relationship. Firstly, the aim of preclinical research needs to be clearly defined. Then you will need to decide what the study will measure, the technique and equipment, and the statistical method that will be applied.

Pilot study: A pilot study is necessary to determine the drug doses, toxicity, incubation time, and logistics. In a rodent study, for example, you may include both sexes, but it is acceptable to work on one sex first if there is a constraint on the resource. Before concluding, the outcomes from preclinical studies require clinical trials to approve efficacy and toxicity.

Sample Size:

Usually, preclinical studies have a small sample size compared to human studies. The reason is that laboratory animals have fewer variations. A power calculation is used to determine the sample size, considering the alpha value, standard deviation, and effect size of similar works published previously. Usually, a preclinical study could set the significance level "α" at 0.05 and two-tailed. The power of the experiment is at 80%.

Conclusion: At the end of a preclinical study, the researcher may suggest that the findings be tested on people.

Clinical Research

Clinical research includes observational and interventional or experimental studies. Observational studies are non-experimental, generating essential insights regarding a medical condition or disease, but cannot conclude cause-and-effect relationships. Human trials or experimental studies are interventional studies that may produce high-quality data and determine cause-effect relationships. An observational study examines the exposure and outcome, while an experimental study investigates an assigned exposure causing the result.

Clinical research: Clinical trials have four phases, each with a unique objective, design, and sample size.

Phases	
I	Test the intervention in healthy volunteers (~100 participants over two years). The goal is to address safety issues, pharmacokinetics, and dose-response characteristics.
II	To determine the evidence of activity and optimal dose (~300 patients up to three years).
III	To provide data for approval by authorities investigating new treatment against placebo or conventional therapy for better outcomes (>1000 patients over three to four years).
IV	To evaluates long-term safety data.

PICOT

PICOT stands for *patient, intervention, comparison, outcome,* and *time.* It can represent the elements of a clinical research question. For example, PICOT can be criteria reviewed when the questions are about therapy, prevention, diagnosis, etiology, and prognosis. You could ask the following:

- *Patients or population problems:* What is the disease or condition, and what are the effects of age, gender, and clinical characteristics?

- *Intervention:* What are the proposed treatments: new drugs, diet, exercise protocol? What are the specific tests?
- *Comparison:* Has an appropriate control group been used? What is the alternative to the intervention?
- *Outcome:* What are the expected results? An improved treatment could lead to better patient outcomes or complete recovery.
- *Time:* Is the time frame a single time point or over several time points, and for how long?

Open, Single-Blind, and Double-Blind Trial

A clinical trial can be an open-label trial, single-blind trial, or double-blind trial. *Blind* means confidentiality in the study design. Furthermore, these studies can be either randomized or non-randomized trials. Also, the studies can be controlled or uncontrolled. An *uncontrolled trial* means there is no placebo group and all participants are on the same treatment.

An Open Trial:

An *open trial,* or *open-label study,* is a study in which both the researcher and participants know the treatment being given. It does not withhold information from the participants and researchers involved in the study. An open trial can be either with or without randomization of participant allocations.

The Single-Blind Trial:

A clinical trial usually has two groups, the treatment group and a control or placebo group. A single-blind trial is where the participants do not know what treatment they receive. This design can reduce the risk of error because some participants might produce fake outcomes if they knew what treatment they were on. However, the researchers know which participants are on the placebo or the treatment. Here, you may find an example of a single-blind randomized controlled trial: "Rationale and Design of a Single-Blind Randomized Controlled Trial of Exercise Training for Managing Learning and Memory Impairment in Persons with Multiple Sclerosis" (Sandroff et al., 2018).

The Double-Blind Trial:

The best clinical research model is a *double-blind trial.* In this model, the participants and researchers do not know which group is on placebo or treatment. It means that (1) participants do not know if they are in the treatment or the placebo group, (2) participants do not know the independent variable or dependent variable, and (3) researchers do not know the independent variable or dependent variable.

The advantage is this model avoids results produced by the placebo effect and researcher bias. Since the participants do not know which group they are in, the risk of spurious results is minimum. On the other hand, the researchers do not know which group the participant is in, and the risk of researcher bias is low. Both make the investigation more accurate.

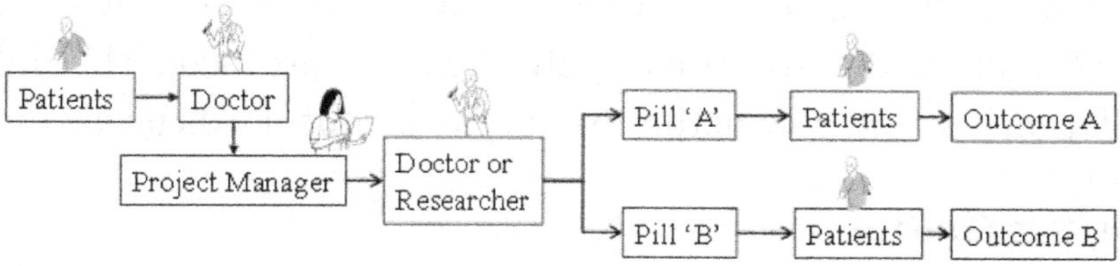

The figure shows the process of a double-blind trial. Patients come to see a doctor for medical conditions. The doctor interviews patients and determines if the patient is suitable for the study and consents to the study. Then, the doctor will ask the project manager. The project manager will confirm, "Yes, Doctor, your patient is eligible for the trial." This patient will be allocated the treatment pack "pill A" without labeling the drug's name. After the trial, the project manager will decode what "pill A" was.

Experimental Control Group

A *control group* is an independent group from the testing group; therefore, the testing variable cannot influence the control group's outcomes. The aim is to eliminate alternative interpretations of the experimental results. A control group is not essential for all medical experiments, but controls are critical to studies with many variations that are challenging to isolate.

Negative Control:

A control group is one that the researcher does not expect to affect the results of an experiment. The *negative control* aims to confirm the testing variable by comparison or whether the effect was caused by some other (possibly unforeseen) variables.

For example, the researcher tests whether an exercise protocol lowers body weight. The negative control would be the group without applying the exercise protocol but under the same conditions as the group using the exercise protocol. The only difference would be whether or not the protocol was used.

Positive Control:

A *positive control* is a control that the researcher knows works.

For example, suppose researchers test a new anti-diabetic drug for type 2 diabetes patients. They could use metformin as the positive control and conduct experiments to evaluate the anti-diabetic effect of the new anti-diabetic drug. Metformin is the experiment's control group and is a positive control because the researchers know how it works.

Placebo Control:

The control avoids possible placebo effects in an experiment. A placebo effect is when the control group participant feels an impact while not being subjected to the treatment. The placebo effect can lead to inaccurate outcomes.

Example: A doctor testing an antidepressant might give the placebo group a pill that doesn't contain any antidepressant but looks identical to the pill given to the experimental group. A placebo pill may show a possible psychological effect instead of the antidepressant effect.

Randomized Control:

This type of control helps to balance the subject variations and makes these variations unpredictable. Therefore, this randomized control is suitable for the participants possessing significant variables.

Example: A researcher recruited 150 subjects to participate in a weight-reduction study. The researchers found considerable body weight and height variations when measuring the baseline demographic information before the intervention trial. In this case, the researcher has decided to use the randomized control method in participant group allocation. If you have taken the baseline variations in the research design, you have introduced bias.

ASK YOURSELF
▪ What is in vitro research? ▪ What is in vitro research? ▪ What are the primary purposes of preclinical research? ▪ What are the four phases of clinical research? ▪ What does PICOT mean? ▪ What is the meaning of *open trial*? ▪ What is the meaning of single-blind trial or double-blind trial? ▪ What is the meaning of negative control, positive control, placebo, or randomized control?

Research Design for Specific Questions

TOPIC OUTLINE
Risk factors
Biomarkers
Prevalence
Diagnosis
Prognosis

Risk Factors

Risk factors for health are the attributes increasing the chances of health harm. You can use either a case-control study or a cohort study to investigate risk factors.

A case-control study can address and identify possible risk factors, particularly suitable for a rare or uncommon disease or a long latency period. The reason is that the observer or researcher starts with a known condition or disease and studies baseline data before the disease develops. The study can use a relatively small sample size and evaluate multiple risk factors. The downside of a case-control study is that it does not determine causality. The reason is that there are chances of recall bias, which can mislead the study's outcomes. A case-control study calculates the odds ratio for risk factors but cannot estimate incidences, including risk ratio or risk difference. This is because the researcher starts with the outcome or disease. However, you do not know the total number of people in your population, which is required to calculate incidences, risk ratio, or risk differences.

A cohort study is more powerful than a case-control study in identifying risk factors. Furthermore, a cohort study can also study the possible cause-effect relationship of a disease. For example, researchers look at baseline data for people who did not initially have an illness and how a risk factor has affected the subject's health over time. Researchers can calculate the odd ratio and risk ratio or risk difference from a cohort study because they know the total number of people in your research. Or researchers can develop a hypothesis that a risk factor can lead to the disease. The study will identify the risk factor's baseline and follow up for the disease development.

Biomarkers

Biomarker or *biological marker* refers to the measures indicating what occurs in a cell or organism at a given time.

Biomarkers are objective signs and can be used for disease diagnosis, personalized medication, and surrogate endpoints in clinical research. It differs from the symptoms reported by the patients.

Biomarkers are molecular, histological, radiographical, or physiological features. The biomarkers can be from protein and genetic tests of blood and other tissues, medical imaging findings, physical measurement (e.g., blood pressure and heart rate), and even behavior.

The classification of biomarkers includes normal biological processes, pathogenic processes, and drug responses. A biomarker can be a predictive, prognostic, pharmacodynamic, or surrogate endpoint indicator.

To identify the biomarker, you need to have two parallel groups featuring two contrast status levels, for example, positive versus negative or high versus low (Gosho et al., 2012). The parallel groups can be one independent variable group and another control group or two independent variables. It is essential to have a well-controlled design to eliminate potential bias or confounding factors.

Prevalence

Prevalence is the proportion of persons with a disease at or during a particular period; therefore, it includes all new and old cases. The calculation is the number of disease cases divided by the total number in a specific population (e.g., %) at a given time. Prevalence can be a point of prevalence or a period of prevalence in a particular population. A cross-sectional design can investigate the prevalence of a health outcome. A cohort study can also be used to calculate the prevalence. For example, the prevalence of overweight and obese Australian adults was 57%, which rose to 66% in 2018. An incidence refers to new cases only, which is different from prevalence.

Diagnosis

A *diagnosis* study refers to a new test contributing to existing tests for a particular disease. A cross-sectional study is a valid study design for estimating the accuracy of diagnosis in a relevant population, while many other methods can also help. For example, you may want to study blood samples, biopsies, colonoscopies, and medical images. Here, the sample size needs to be sufficient for external representation. In addition, the study should avoid any bias and confoundings.

Prognosis

Prognosis refers to what will happen to patients after treatment in the short and long term, for example, quality of life, disease progression, and survival.

For example, the prognosis of breast cancer surgery depends on the cancer stage, patient age, and general condition. The family will want to know how long the patient will live, what kind of life the patient can expect after surgery, and whether the patient is likely to have recurrent cancer. A prognosis study can address these questions. In addition, the prognosis study can help the decision-making for follow-up treatment and care.

The best design for a prognostic study is a cohort study to follow the patients over time with multiple measures. For example, if you want to find out why some patients had depression but not others after the surgery, you can use a cohort study.

Depending on the question, you could also use a case-control study to investigate prognosis-related questions. For example, you can use a case-control study to examine whether smoking affects breast cancer recovery after surgery.

ASK YOURSELF
▪ Why can a risk factor be calculated in case-control and cohort studies? ▪ What are biomarkers used for? ▪ What are the differences between disease prevalence and disease incidence? ▪ Why is a cross-sectional study used for estimating the accuracy of diagnosis? ▪ Why is a cohort study suitable for a prognostic study?

Descriptive Research

TOPIC OUTLINE

- Survey study
- Case report
- Case series study

A *descriptive study* aims to describe population or group characteristics. The frequently asked questions are how, what, when, and where. Next, the researcher collects the data to describe the characteristics of the study variables, such as demographic features, clinical characteristics, conditions, and phenomena. Descriptive research design focuses on observations and measurements but not manipulated variables. Three common descriptive studies are *survey, observational,* and *case* or *case-series reports.*

Survey Study

Here, we introduce four common descriptive survey studies and describe their aims, relevant questions, and examples.

Descriptive Survey

A *descriptive survey* collects the data from participants. For example, a researcher wants to determine the percentage of smokers among schizophrenia patients in a hospital. The researcher uses a survey as the research instrument, and each item on the survey related to smoking is subjected to a yes/no answer.

A Descriptive-Normative Survey

A *descriptive-normative survey* goes beyond the descriptive survey to compare a survey with the norm. For example, you wish to know the rate of smokers in a patient group compared with a non-patient group. You can use a chi-square test to calculate the statistical difference between them. This method frequently appears in a clinical study's demographic and clinical characteristic table.

A Descriptive-Comparative Study

A *descriptive-comparative study* aims to compare two variables to determine whether one is better than another. It does not manipulate the variables or data, meaning it uses a subjective approach. For example, a doctor wants to test two anti-diabetic drugs and determine which one is better for controlling blood glucose levels in diabetic patients. The researcher gives two different anti-diabetic medicines to the patients and compares which one is better. Blood glucose levels, duration of application, and other parameters are subject to evaluation to determine which drug is more effective.

A Descriptive-Status Study

A *descriptive-status study* aims to quantify real-life situations. For example, a researcher investigates the exercise frequency of older people and the relationship with their cognition, e.g., memory scores. The researcher gathers the outcomes of the exercise frequency and memory scores. This research can assist in determining whether more exercise leads to better memory performance, but low or no exercise is associated with lower memory scores or vice versa.

Case Report

A *case report* aims to describe an unusual finding or novel event of a single subject or specific small group with practical or clinical significance. The discovery should be significant and may lead to developing new ideas or hypotheses for follow-up studies. The case report is a brief and quick communication between practitioners or researchers and practitioners.

A typical situation for a case report may be a disease associated with an unexpected symptom, an unusual sign when treating or observing a medical condition, an unexpected side-effect, or a better treatment method.

The structure of a case report should have a title, abstract, literature review, case, discussion, conclusion, and references. The format may vary depending on the different journals you will need to check before submitting a paper for publication.

Title: The title should be informative and precise.

Abstract: The abstract is usually short, about 150 or fewer words. It summarizes the case, issues, and take-home message.

Introduction: The introduction should state the problem to be addressed, justify why to report the case, and summarize relevant literature.

Case: The case can include the history, examination methods, treatment, and outcomes.

Discussion: The discussion can start by synchronizing and pointing out the introduction's highlights and then focusing on novelty and meaning or interpretation of the results. This section should provide the existing knowledge and relevant findings on the critical issues. Next, the discussion should point out the area of disparities or research gaps. Finally, the report may connect what we know, the new findings, and how the discovery adds to the existing literature.

Conclusion: The report ends with summary points. It should provide readers with the take-home message, limitations, and implications and point out future research direction.

Informed consent is mandatory for a case report and is usually requested by publishers. Patient anonymity ensures the confidentiality of personal privacy. Do not publish patients' photos.

Figures and tables can help the presentation by highlighting the discoveries and summarizing data.

References: Relevant literature cited in the report should be listed at the end of the paper.

Example: A Pilot Study to Generate a New Hypothesis

Here is an example of a case report. Olanzapine is an antipsychotic drug frequently used for treating schizophrenia. However, it can cause severe weight gain, obesity, and metabolic syndrome. So researchers launched a pilot study using an anti-obesity drug, lorcaserin, to counteract antipsychotic drug-induced obesity in *two* patients (Nguyen et al., 2015). Since there were only two patients, it is a pilot study. In this study, researchers measured metabolic parameters, including the baseline, three months, and fourteen months after the treatments. The outcome showed that lorcaserin prevented excessive weight gain and improved lipid profiles for the patients. Therefore, the researchers suggest that lorcaserin may help to reduce obesity, while a large clinical study is required.

Case-Series Study

A *case series* is a descriptive and observational study, usually in a clinical or practical situation. This type of study reports multiple cases having the same symptom. Therefore, clinical samples should be representative of a clinical population. The study can lead to a hypothesis for a new study.

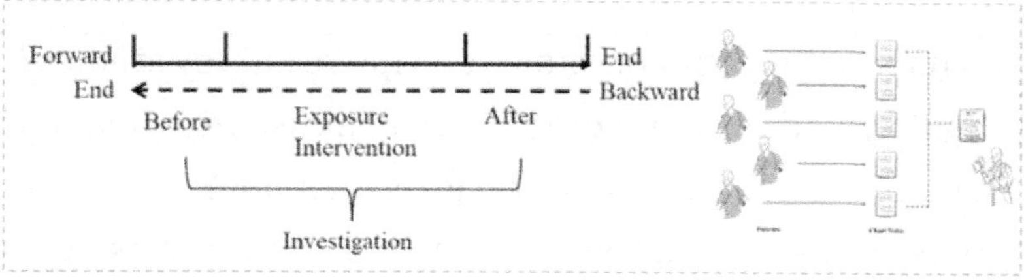

Forward-looking: A case-series study may follow the patients exposed to a condition, intervene, or investigate the patients before and after the exposure.

Backward-looking: Researchers can investigate subjects with the same disease and then analyze previous exposure data.

Although a case-series study is similar to a cohort study, it usually does not have a control group (Mathes and Pieper, 2017). Sometimes, it is also called a *self-controlled case-series study*.

A case-series study cannot inform a cause-effect relationship.

Example: To Reveal the Confounder for Drug Resistance

Here is an example of a case-series study. Depression patients often have vitamin D deficiency (possible confounder). Both depression and vitamin D can cause somatic symptoms, such as fatigue, body pains, and unrefreshing sleep. Therefore, depressant-resistance in some patients could be due to vitamin D deficiency. If it is, supplementation of vitamin D will help the treatment. Researchers recruited sixty-two depression patients and screened them for vitamin D deficiency. Vitamin D deficient patients were prescribed vitamin D to relieve somatic symptoms (Nadkarni and Odejayi, 2014). As a case-series study, it generated some interesting findings; however, it needs a more extensive and appropriately designed study before concluding.

ASK YOURSELF
▪ What are the four common descriptive survey studies? ▪ Could you describe the structure of a case report study? ▪ What is the definition of a case-series study? ▪ Why can a case-series study not inform a cause-effect relationship?

Observational and Correlational Research

TOPIC OUTLINE

- Cross-sectional study
- Case-control study
- Cohort study

An *observational study* aims to describe one or a set of variables by observations. Observations may include the effect of a risk factor exposure, diagnostic test, and intervention without changing any exposure factors or the participant information. The research questions are the difference, association, risk factor, or prevalence.

Qualitative Observational Study

The *qualitative observational study* aims to collect data and generate multiple answers using subjective methodologies. The study is objective, conducted with a small sample, counted as the actual, and portrays an individual opinion. For example, a doctor wants to understand why schizophrenia patients often do not comply with chronic antipsychotic medication. Others like to study the taste (bitter or sweet), mood (happy or depressed), and texture (rough and smooth).

Quantitative Observational Study

The *quantitative observational study* aims to measure the variables using numerical and statistical methods objectively. Therefore, it is about quantitative measures such as weight, length, age, distance, temperature, and scale. For example, the blood glucose level is 5.5 mmol/L. This type of study is subjective, has a large sample, and is a collection of outcomes in numbers. It can be a cross-sectional, case-control, or cohort study.

Correlational Study

A correlational study aims to investigate relationships between variables without data manipulation. It reflects strength and direction, such as *r* value and positive, negative, or no correlations. It belongs to a non-experimental design, meaning no extraneous variables on the variables under study. The study design includes observational, archival (e.g., cross-sectional and case-control), and survey studies.

Cross-Sectional Study

A *cross-sectional study* belongs to observational research at one specific point in time. The style is descriptive and analytical. However, it is neither a longitudinal nor an experimental study. Therefore, it is also known as a *cross-sectional analysis, transversal research*, or *prevalence study*.

It is frequently used in medical and social science research to determine the differences and relationships between variables and establish diagnostic criteria. It involves analyzing data collected from a population or a representative subset of subjects.

Here are examples of two cross-sectional studies.

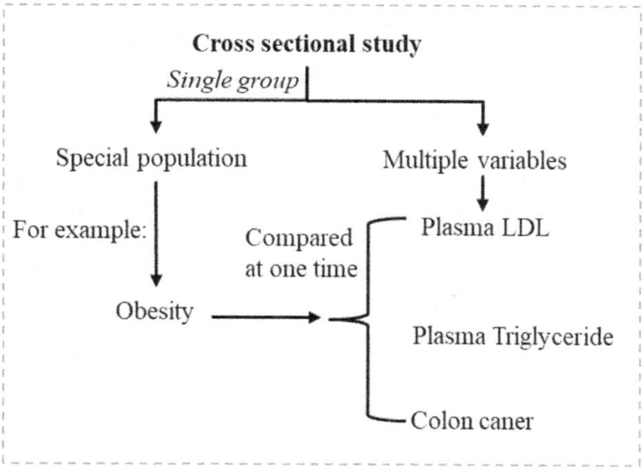

The figure shows a single-group cross-sectional study investigating a particular population on multiple variables. For example, obese subjects could have an elevated plasma low-density lipoprotein (LDL, > 1.8 mmol/l) and triglyceride (> 2.0 mmol/l) and an increased incidence of colon cancer. Researchers can design a cross-sectional study, collect data at a specific time, and perform correlation analysis.

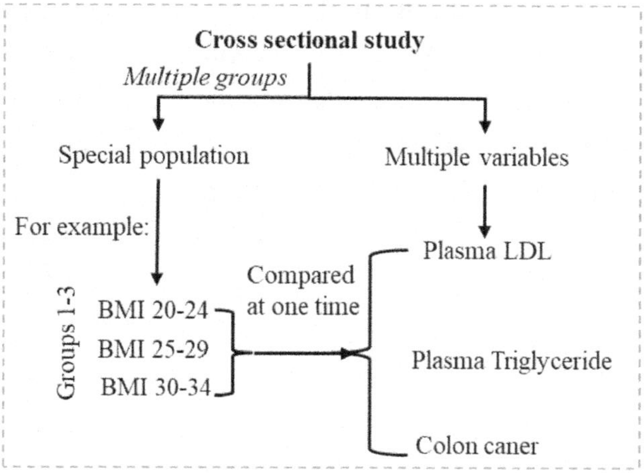

The figure shows a multiple-group cross-sectional study having several groups from a particular population with multiple variables measured. For example, three groups are the subjects having normal body weight (BMI from 20 to 24), overweight (BMI from 25 to 29), and obese (BMI from 30 to 34). As a cross-sectional study, researchers collected multiple variables from these subjects, for example, LDL, triglyceride, and incidence of colon cancer. The research design can use analysis of variance to determine the differences between groups and correlation analysis to show multiple variable relationships.

Example 1: You Can Use a Cross-Sectional Study to Determine the Relationship Between Variables Assisting Diagnosis

Bodyweight alone is inappropriate for diagnosing obesity because height contributes to body weight. Therefore, body mass index (BMI) is a more appropriate indicator for diagnosing obesity. BMI is a calculation of BMI = kg/m^2, body weight in kg divided by height square in meters. Obesity is an excessive body fat deposition that increases the health risk for several diseases. Therefore, an appropriate diagnostic criterion is essential. A correlation analysis between BMI and body fat will help the establishment of BMI as an obesity indicator. A single group cross-sectional study can examine such a relationship. The independent variable BMI and the dependent variable (body fat percentage) can be continuous variables.

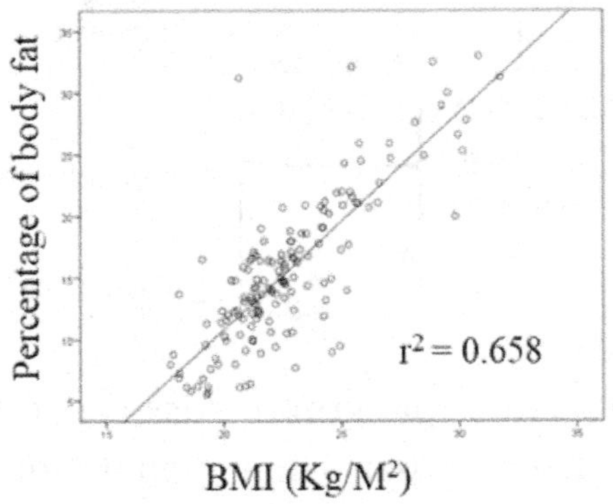

The figure shows the two variables in a cross-sectional study. BMI and body fat percentage correlation is $r^2 = 0.658$ or 66%, which is a strong correlation. Therefore, BMI can be an indicator of obesity, although there can be more. For example, waist circumference is another indicator of obesity (That is, women: > 88 cm, men: > 102 cm). Since this study has only one group of participants, the external validity of the results will rely on where the sample was from and the size sample; therefore, the interpretation of the results needs to be cautious.

Example 2: You Can Use a Cross-Sectional Study with Linear Regression Analysis to Identify a Predictor

Chronic low-grade inflammation can affect cognition. C-reactive protein (CRP) is a protein molecule made by the liver and secreted into the circulation. It is an indicator of systematic inflammation. The low risk of heart disease is < 2 mg/L, and the high risk is ≥ 2 mg/L. Researchers want to know if CRP levels predict cognitive function. Therefore, this question requires an association study to calculate the β coefficient. The research design can be a single-group cross-sectional study having multiple outcome variables. A linear regression equation uses CRP to predict cognition scores based on the β value. An example of a study (Vintimilla et al., 2019) showed a significant regression equation in 328 participants with high CRP levels for verbal fluency scores, $F_{(1\text{-}327)} = 4.59$, $p = 0.03$ and increased CRP can predict verbal fluency scores, $\beta = -0.135$, $p = 0.01$. It means that for every one mg/L CRP increase in this population, the prediction is that there is a corresponding decrease in verbal fluency score by 0.135.

Example 3: You Can Use a Cross-Sectional Study with Logistic Regression Analysis to Determine the Risk Factor

Aging is associated with declined cognitive function and chronic low-grade inflammation. Researchers want to determine if chronic low-grade inflammation is a risk factor for cognitive decline. Determination of a risk factor requires an association study by calculating OR values. For example, the researchers recruited 329 subjects and counted the number of subjects by their low and high CRP scores and their low and normal cognitive function scores (Vintimilla et al., 2019). Logistic regression analysis showed that OR is 1.75 (95% CI = 1.13 - 2.72, $p = 0.01$). A high CRP score gave 1.75 times higher risk of low cognitive function.

Example 4: A Cross-Sectional Study Needs to Control for Confounders

A human study with a large sample size can have multiple covariates. Usually, cross-sectional research requires a large sample size of more than two hundred subjects. The covariates can be age, gender, education level, and medical history, affecting the outcome variables. In addition, the research design should set the inclusion and exclusion criteria and remove unnecessary confounders.

A cross-sectional study may need a longitudinal study to confirm the findings. For example, at the end of a cross-sectional study, the author may suggest a population's longitudinal analysis to explain further the relationship between CRP concentrations and cognitive functioning mentioned in example 3 above. Would you be able to explain why this should be the case?

Example 5: Evidence Strength Comparing Case-Report and Cross-Section Studies

A case-series study reported that dining in a restaurant near the beach caused customers to get food poisoning. It is questionable to have a conclusion as such. The evidence of food poisoning cannot be taken as a permanent fact because it is not immutable or incapable of change. Changing practices at the restaurant will decrease food poisoning, leading to a change in the evidence. So the concept cannot be extended to say, "Eating in this restaurant will make you sick."

In contrast, in a *cross-sectional* study where a hospital examines, for example, one thousand patients and finds a high prevalence of cardiovascular disease in older people, the evidence is more reliable based on a larger sample size than in a case-series study. You could consider this evidence that age contributes to cardiovascular disease because it is based on an established form of scientific research and not simply on the observation of several persons.

Case-Control Study

A case-control study compares subjects with a disease of interest (cases) with those without a disease (controls). It looks retrospectively to examine how frequently the exposure to a risk factor is present in each group to determine the relationship between the risk factor and the disease. Unfortunately, case-control studies often rely on people trying to recall past symptoms or lifestyle factors, thus limiting their scientific value.

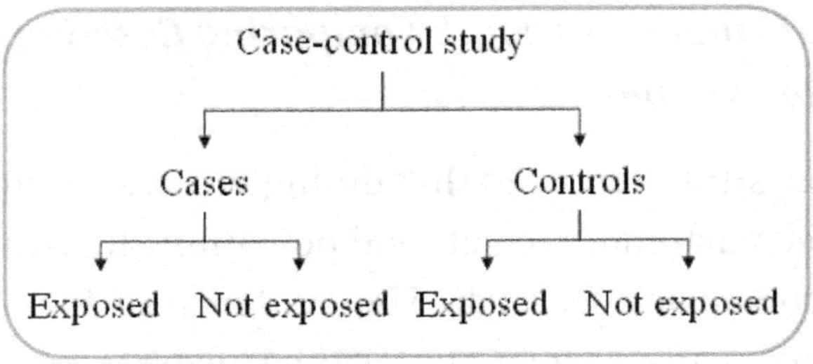

The flowchart shows a standard design for a case-control study. It compares the frequency between exposure and non-exposure to a risk factor to determine the relationship between the risk factor and the disease.

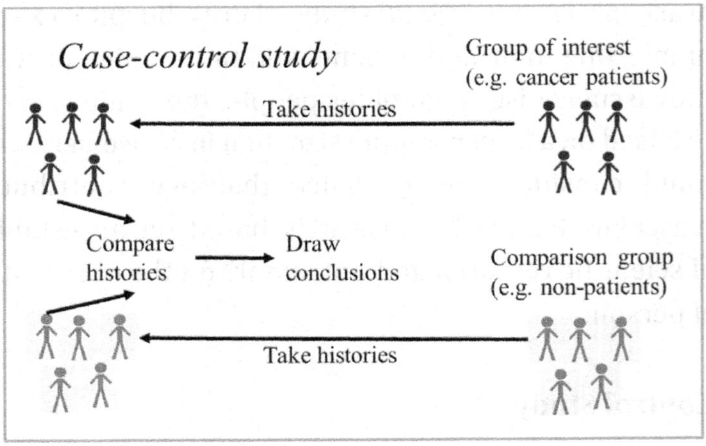

The figure shows a known disease. The researcher wants to find the risk factor. For example, a group of subjects with lung cancer and another group without lung cancer, controls, are asked to recall their past experiences. Researchers compare the retrospective histories of both groups and the data to determine possible risk factors. It is noted that the scientific value of case-control studies is limited because they rely on memories that may sometimes be inaccurate.

Features of a Case-Control Study

- It belongs to an observational study.
- There is no intervention involved.
- No attempt aims to alter the course of the disease.
- The risk factor is retrospectively determined.
- You can report the odds ratio or relative risk value.

Advantages of a Case-Control Study

- Efficiency is an advantage of a case-control study, requiring less time and resources.
- For rare diseases as it can be performed based on a smaller sample size compared with a cross-sectional study.
- It allows multiple risk factors to be examined simultaneously.
- You can use this study to establish the relationship between the variables of your interest and generate hypotheses for further investigation.

Disadvantages of a Case-Control Study

- Susceptible to bias since the data rely on the subjects' memories, which can be inaccurate.
- Prone to methodological errors because it is not a pre-designed study.
- It works only under certain types of conditions because it is retrospective.
- It could be challenging to find a suitable control group. You have to work under certain conditions.

- It belongs to the observational study and does not address the cause-effect relationship.
- The design is different between a case-series study and a case-control study. Case series have no control group as the study recruits patients only. However, a case-control study does require the control group, which is another group of, for example, healthy individuals, a different disease, or self-control (e.g., crossover design).

Example 1: You Can Use a Case-Control Study to Investigate the Risk Factor or OR Value

Metabolic syndrome is a cluster of metabolic conditions increasing the risks for type 2 diabetes, cardiovascular disease, and cognitive decline. Bipolar patients often have an elevated blood uric acid level or hyperuricemia and a high incidence of metabolic syndrome. Therefore, we want to investigate if hyperuricemia is associated with metabolic syndrome in bipolar patients (Chen et al., 2018). The question is about the relationship between hyperuricemia and metabolic syndrome; therefore, we designed a case-control study. We recruited the patients with bipolar disorder and healthy controls with or without metabolic syndrome; hence, there were four groups. We measured the blood uric acid in all four groups. Researchers calculated OR to determine if hyperuricemia is a risk factor for metabolic syndrome in bipolar patients. The analysis included 318 bipolar patients and 160 healthy controls. The results showed hyperuricemia was associated with metabolic syndrome in bipolar patients ($p < 0.001$). Bipolar patients who developed metabolic syndrome had an increased prevalence of hyperuricemia OR = 3.0, 95% CI, 1.7 - 5.4.

Example 2: Using the Chi-Square Test in a Case-Control Study, You Can Analyze the Nominal Baseline Data

We investigated whether or not hyperuricemia is associated with metabolic syndrome. First, we analyzed the baseline differences of potential confounding factors for metabolic syndrome between the patient and control groups. Since the data were nominal, a chi-square test was used to examine the observed results (disease) with expected results (e.g., patients versus controls). We found no statistical difference in gender and marital status, both $p > 0.05$; however, there were significant differences in smokers, $p < 0.05$ (Chen et al., 2018). Therefore, smoking should be checked for being a possible confounder associated with metabolic syndrome.

Example 3: You Can Use a Case-Control Study to Investigate a Disease Risk Factor

A cross-sectional study shows that sun exposure is associated with all skin cancers. However, we do not know the relationship between how much and what pattern of sun exposure increases skin cancer (English et al., 1998). A case-control study should be able to address this question. The research design includes recruiting subjects with or without skin cancer. Then, the researcher interviews the subjects about their lifetime sun exposure, e.g., quantity, location, and age. After collecting the data, they calculate the OR value. The result shows that the OR is 3.3 (CI 1.3 - 8.2, $p = 0.01$) at sixty-five thousand hours of sun exposure, meaning a 3.3 times higher risk of developing skin cancer.

Example 4: You Can Use a Case-Control Study to Determine a Possible Interaction Between Two Diseases on One Symptom

Patients may have two health conditions, such as schizophrenia patients with type 2 diabetes. Schizophrenia and diabetes can both affect cognitive function. However, whether the cognitive impairment was due to schizophrenia, diabetes, or a combination of the two is unclear. The research design requires a two-way ANOVA to determine if there is an interaction effect between schizophrenia and diabetes (Han et al., 2013). We found a significant interaction effect between schizophrenia and diabetes on cognitive impairments ($p < 0.01$). To decompose this two-way interaction, we compared language scores separately by healthy controls with and without diabetes and with schizophrenia with and without diabetes. Schizophrenia with and without diabetes had worse cognitive performance ($p < 0.01$) with effect sizes ranging from 0.23 to 0.56. Therefore, schizophrenia with diabetes had more cognitive impairment than schizophrenia without diabetes.

Example 5: Using Logistic Regression to Calculate OR, You Can Use a Case-Control Study to Investigate the Death Risk Factors

Clinical studies of COVID-19 infection showed different clinical and laboratory features between survivors and non-survivors. Therefore, researchers want to investigate the feasible parameters to predict the patient prognosis with COVID-19 disease. The research design includes the discharge and death groups (Pan et al., 2020). Bivariate logistic regression analyzed all variables and identified the parameters significantly associated with death events. Furthermore, a multivariate logistic regression showed a significant model fitting of the critical parameters as independent risk factors with high OR values ($p < 0.04$). The study concluded that systematic inflammation with cardiac dysfunction was likely a primary reason for death events in COVID-19, in addition to acute respiratory distress syndrome.

Cohort Study

A cohort study follows the participants over a set period; therefore, it is longitudinal. The researcher typically observes participants, monitors their exposure to the risk factor, and identifies the disease's possible causal factors. In addition, during this longitudinal study, the researcher can perform cross-sectional studies at specific intervals to calculate the OR values or the risk factors. Therefore, a cohort study can study either association or cause of an outcome between risk factors and disease outcomes.

A cohort study can be used to do the following:

- Investigate the risk factor causing the disease
- Evaluate risk factors, such as rare risk factors
- Establish the link between risk factors and health outcomes

A cohort study is to study a risk factor or treatment where the researcher follows the subjects over time to determine the relationship between the exposure and subsequent outcomes. Furthermore, a cohort study requires a control group without exposure to the risk.

When designing a cohort study, it is essential to control potential bias and confoundings.

If subjects already had the disease, they would not be suitable for a cohort study.

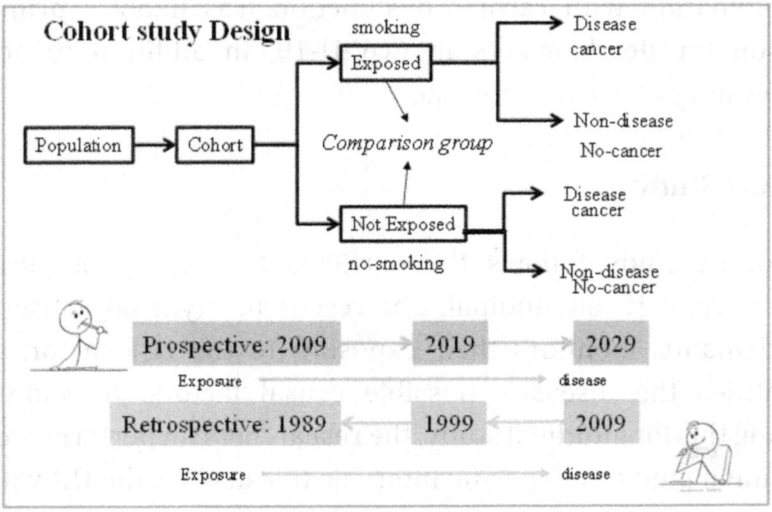

The figure shows that a cohort study can establish the link between a risk factor and health outcomes. The research follows the subjects to determine a disease outcome. It can be either a prospective or retrospective study.

Prospective Cohort Study

The researcher can plan and design a prospective cohort study in advance. The flowchart above shows that the researcher on the top row will perform a prospective cohort study from left to right. The first group of subjects had exposure to the risk factor (e.g., smoking), while the second group did not expose to the risk factor (e.g., no smoking). The outcomes (e.g., lung cancer) will be recorded regularly during the study, for example, every second year. After several years, the researcher will have recorded the number of participants who developed the disease (lung cancer) and participants who did not.

Retrospective Cohort Study

The researchers perform the study based on the data already collected in a database that will be a retrospective cohort study. The flowchart above shows that the researcher conducts a retrospective cohort study on the bottom row. The study will have two subject groups. Group one was exposed to the risk factor, but group two was not exposed to the risk factor. Disease occurrences are identified from each group. In this case, the researcher cannot go back and regain missing data because the study is retrospective; therefore, the interpretation is limited.

The Population of a Cohort Study

A general population or a specific subject group is suitable for a cohort study, depending on how you want to generalize the findings.

For example, the Framingham heart study investigates the residents of Framingham City, Massachusetts, USA. This ongoing long-term cardiovascular cohort study began in 1948 with over five thousand subjects for several decades.

A specific subject group or a rare disease study could be recruited for the above population to examine a risk factor. For example, the Nurses' Health Study examines the long-term effects of the environment on health and disease development. The research design may control potential bias and confounding factors if it is a prospective cohort study.

Basic Procedures of a Cohort Study

Enrollment: Enroll the subjects at risk and investigate the disease development. These subjects should not have that disease at the start of the study. The researcher plans the study and monitors the research over a set period.

Measure outcomes: The research measures the health outcomes (e.g., disease) over time, which could be several measurements with regular intervals.

Analysis: The researcher analyses risk factors and reports outcomes based on collected data. In a cohort study, the analysis can include the risk ratio, risk difference, relative risk, or odds ratio.

Example 1: You Can Use a Cohort Study to Estimate the Risk Using a Hazard Regression Analysis

Sunscreen use has protective effects on reducing melanoma risk; however, it depends on whether sunscreen has a low or high sun protection factor (SPF). A researcher hypothesized that sunscreen use is related to melanoma risk, and low and high SPF differ in protection when sunbathing. The question is suitable for a cohort study. The study design involves previous and newly collected data retrospectively and prospectively. Here, the duration was from one to sixteen years. The independent variables were the low and high SPF sunscreens. The outcome variable was melanoma. Multivariable Cox proportional hazards regression estimated the association between sunscreen use and melanoma risk by calculating hazard ratios and 95% CI. The analysis showed that SPF $\geq$ 15 sunscreen reduces melanoma risk in a sizeable population (Ghiasvand et al., 2016).

Example 2: A Cohort Study Is a Longitudinal Study and Can Last for Decades

The Framingham Heart Study investigates population health to unravel patterns applied to the general population to improve the "generalizability" of results. This study began in 1948 with 5,209 adult subjects and is now on its third generation of participants. It is a long-term, ongoing cohort study of Framingham residents and covers many longitudinal studies. It investigated the epidemiology of hypertension, arteriosclerotic cardiovascular disease, and other conditions influenced by diet, exercise, and common medications.

The Framingham Study has produced many significant discoveries.

- The 1960s: Cigarette smoking and obesity increase the risk of heart disease, while exercise decreases it.
- The 1970s: Elevated blood pressure increases the risk of stroke. Psychosocial factors affect the risk of heart disease.
- The 1980s: High HDL cholesterol levels reduce the risk of heart disease.
- The 1990s: Having an enlarged left ventricle of the heart increases the risk of stroke. Elevated blood pressure can progress to heart failure.
- The 2000s: Obesity is a risk factor for heart failure. Serum aldosterone levels predict the risk of elevated blood pressure. Some genes increase the risk of atrial fibrillation. The risk of poor memory is increased in middle-aged men and women if either of their parents has dementia.

Case-Control Versus Cohort Study

In a case-control study, the researcher does not know the exposure, starts with a known disease, and determines the risk factor.

In a cohort study, the researcher studies the risk factor and determines the disease's causal factor.

Table: Similarity and difference between case-control and cohort studies

Case-control study	Cohort study
Retrospective	Prospective or retrospective
Known disease, study *association* with risk factor	Known risk factor; determine the *causal role* contributing to the disease
Weak evidence	Strong evidence
Study association	Can study the causal effect
Other differences	
Rare disease	Rare exposures
Multiple exposures	Multiple outcomes
Less time consuming	Time-consuming
Inexpensive	Expensive

ASK YOURSELF
▪ What is the definition of a cross-sectional study? ▪ What is the definition of a case-control study? ▪ How many groups should a standard case-control study have? ▪ What are the characteristics of a case-control study? ▪ What are the aims of a cohort study? ▪ What are the main procedures of a cohort study? ▪ What are the similarities and differences between a retrospective and prospective cohort study? ▪ What are the differences between a case-control study and a cohort study?

Randomized Controlled Trial

TOPIC OUTLINE
▪ Sample randomization ▪ True experimental design ▪ Quasi-experimental design ▪ Types of quasi-experimental design ▪ One-group pretest-posttest design ▪ Two-group pretest-posttest design ▪ One-way repeated measures design ▪ Steps of a randomized controlled trial

What Is a Randomized Controlled Trial?

A randomized controlled trial (RCT) is a clinical intervention study where the researcher randomly assigns the participants to one of the study groups, i.e., the intervention group and the control group. The intervention group receives the treatment, and the control or comparison group receives an alternative treatment.

The Primary Aim of an RCT Is as Follows:

- Establish cause-effect relationships
- Determine which treatment is superior among competing treatments or control
- Eliminate selection bias
- Avoid confounding factors

RCT is the best experimental or intervention study to investigate a new therapy's efficacy and safety. It is because subjects are allocated randomly (by chance alone), thus minimizing possible bias.

The Advantages of an RCT Are as Follows:

- Randomization reduces possible bias.
- It is easier to blind/mask than observational studies.
- Researchers can analyze the data with well-known statistical tools.
- Populations of participating individuals are clearly identified and randomly allocated.
- When is an RCT useful? When there is a large sample size and measurable dependent variables.

Disadvantages of an RCT Trial Are as Follows:

- It is expensive in terms of time and cost.
- There is always a possibility of losing subjects.
- It is not applicable when the sample size is small and hard to measure or there are diverse outcomes.
- It is not suitable for a quick answer.

Sample Randomization

Random sampling is when researchers randomly allocate participants into groups. It aims to reduce study bias. Randomization doesn't necessarily mean a blind study.

Simple Randomization:

Simple randomization is based on a single sequence of random assignments. Practically, you can flip a coin or throw dice. Also, you can use a statistics book or a computer to generate a number for sample allocation. Simple randomization requires a large sample size to produce groups of the same or similar size; therefore, it is not suitable for a small sample size, which would result in an unequal number of participants among groups. A large clinical trial may use a simple randomization design with a sample size greater than one hundred (Suresh, 2011).

Block Randomization:

Block randomization is suitable for a clinical trial with a small to medium sample size of less than one hundred. You may allocate the participants into randomized groups of equal sample size (table below). The table shows four groups or blocks of participants. Blocks are small and balanced with predesigned arrangements. The aim is to avoid imported differences between groups by chance (Vickers, 2006).

Table: Block randomization assignment

Round	Group 1	Group 2	Group 3	Group 4
1	Intervention	Intervention	Control	Control
2	Intervention	Control	Intervention	Control
3	Intervention	Control	Control	Intervention
4	Control	Control	Intervention	Intervention
5	Control	Intervention	Control	Intervention
6	Control	Intervention	Intervention	Control
...				

Stratified Randomization:

Stratified randomization aims to control the influence of covariates by balancing the baseline characteristics or covariates. First, the researcher needs to identify possible covariates on the dependent variables. After assigning participants into blocks, simple randomization is performed within each block. For example, age could be a confounding variable and affect the results. Stratified randomization can balance such variations in blocks. The procedure can refer to the block randomization table.

Adaptive Covariate Randomization:

Adaptive covariate randomization assigns a new participant to the specific covariate group, minimizing imbalance in particular covariates (Vickers, 2006).

The table shows adaptive covariate randomization		
Variable	Intervention	Control
Total number of patients	33	44
Back pain	12 (36%)	13 (30%)
Head pain	13(39%)	11 (25%)
Use pain killer	5 (15%)	11 (25%)
Use opiates	3 (9%)	9 (20%)

Procedures of an RCT

Enrollment:

Although there are many retrospective registrations, an RCT prefers to have a prospective registration. The advantage is that the registration allows public scrutiny of the trials, facilitates the exposure of study gaps, and avoids repetition. The World Health Organization considers that the registration of all intervention studies is "a scientific, ethical, and moral responsibility."

Researchers need to decide the study population and gain ethical approval, followed by participant recruitment, eligibility screening, and inclusion and exclusion assessments as a starting procedure.

Researchers may record baseline data, such as demographic data and clinical characteristics.

Allocation:

Participants are allocated randomly into a treatment or control group by chance without the say of the researchers or regard for the participants' preference.

Baseline Data:

Researchers should not analyze baseline differences in an RCT because it could introduce bias. This claim is under the assumption of a large sample size, for example, in hundreds or thousands, where the data between the groups should be similar. However, the baseline data is unlikely to be equal when the sample size is small. In this case, the testing effect may not show because of variations in the baseline data. Another way to avoid possible baseline confounders is to use a repeated measurement design which is very powerful in discovering the intervention effect.

Follow-Up Study:

A follow-up study aims to monitor the participant's health over time after treatment. Timewise, the measurements can be during, at the end, or after the intervention. Researchers can measure the outcome variables in the treatment and control groups at various stages. Furthermore, researchers should record how many participants dropped out and what unexpected situations occurred during the study.

RCT Data Analysis:

There are two analyses commonly used in an RCT.

Intention-to-treat (ITT) analysis: ITT analysis includes all patients randomized in the trial. Based on this definition, the patients who are non-compliant with the treatment or control and drop out prematurely should be included in the ITT analysis. The outcome can be some patients in the treatment group who had no treatment or data (dropouts).

Per-protocol (PP) analysis: PP analysis includes only those patients who adhered to the protocol and completed the treatment allocated initially. The aim is to identify a treatment outcome occurring under optimal conditions.

Usually, an RCT reports both ITT and PP analyses. If doing PP only, the study may have included bias.

The ITT and PP are valid analysis methods in an RCT. The strength of ITT is to reduce possible bias.

Here we have two questions for you.

- Which analysis is the more conservative or under-estimate an effect between ITT and PP analyses?
- What analysis should be used to investigate the effect if participants are fully compliant?

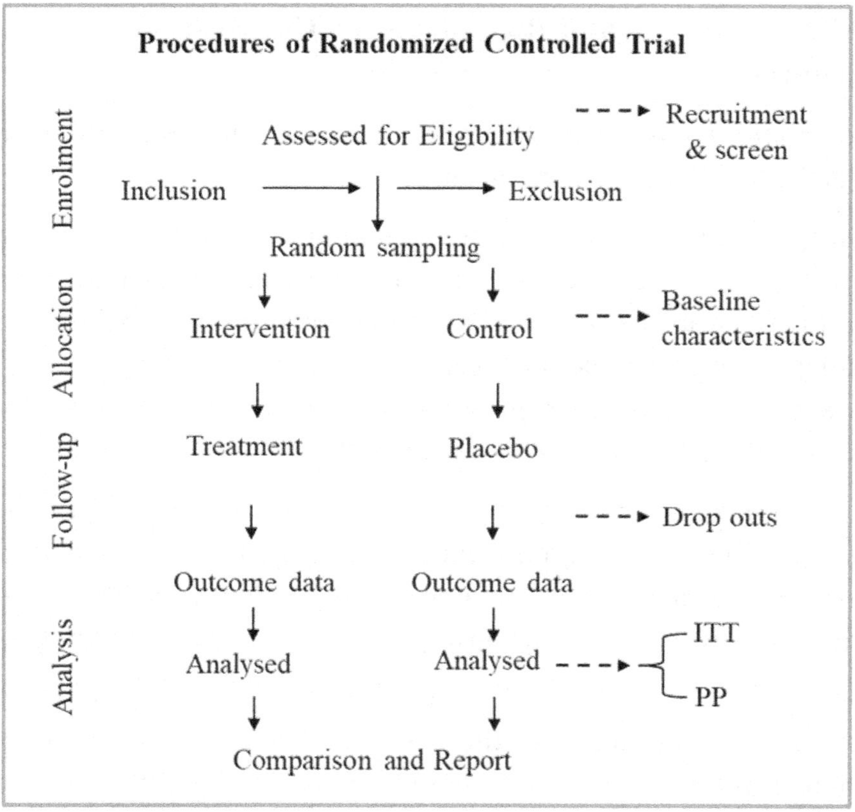

An RCT should follow the above Consolidated Standards of Reporting Trials (CONSORT) guideline.

A True Experimental Design

A true experimental design establishes the cause-effect relationship between variables. It is a robust design that can generate evidence to support a causal and consequence relationship between the independent and outcome variables.

A True Experimental Study Requires Three Essential Criteria

Random assignment: Researchers randomly allocate the participants into research groups.

Independent variable: The independent variable is a known challenge, for example, a treatment that influences the outcomes of other variables. Researchers can control or manipulate the independent variable and observe the outcome variables. For example, a researcher provides the treatment, followed by observations of the effects caused by the treatment.

Control group: At least one control group and one treatment group. The control group aims to control the effects of the extraneous variable on outcome variables. Control subjects are similar to the experimental group in number and characteristics.

An ideal situation would be that there were no significant baseline differences in the total number of participants, demographics, and clinical characteristics between the control and treatment groups.

A Two-Arm RCT

Two-arm RCT is the most often used research design. Researchers randomly assign the participants into two groups, comparing the effects of the treatment group with those of the control group. A two-armed design, also known as a *separate-arm trial,* has one control group per intervention.

This type of design is simple and flexible, and can be performed over a short period. In addition, a two-arm trial is relatively easy to manage compared to a multi-arm trial. Therefore, it is suitable for a more focused study with existing pilot work and substantial evidence.

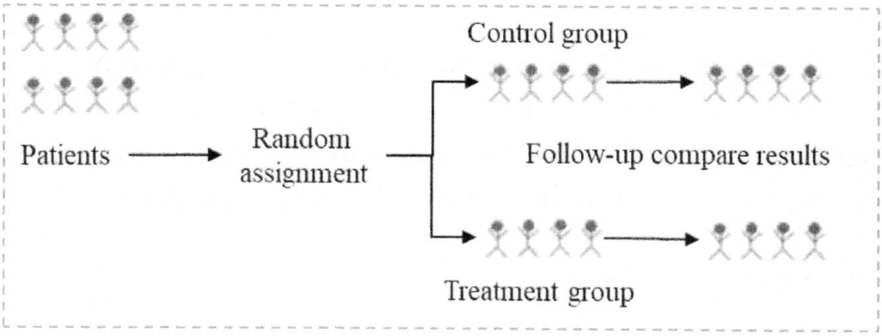

The figure shows a two-arm RCT. First, random assignment allocates the patients into either a control or treatment group receiving a placebo or treatment. Then, the researcher collects and analyzes the data at the end of the trial.

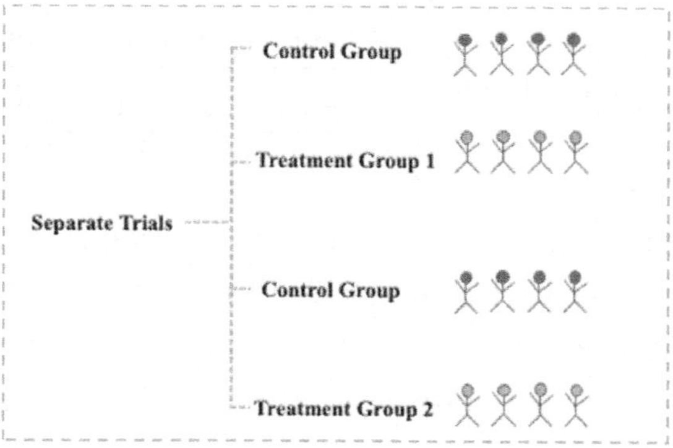

The figure shows another design of a two-arm RCT. In this design, there are separate trials grouped. Here, you have four groups, including two control groups; however, these are two two-arm RCTs running in parallel.

What Are the Common Types of True Experimental Design?

The standard true experimental designs are:

- Posttest only design
- Pretest and posttest design

In addition, among the above two designs, you can use multiple measurements after the first outcome, which is an extended-level design. Also, you can use a crossover design within these true experimental designs, which will be described below.

A Posttest-Only Design

Researchers randomly assign the participants into two groups, receiving either control or treatment. The outcome of variables is measured once after the treatment. The outcome comparisons are then made between the control and treatment groups. There is no measurement before the treatment.

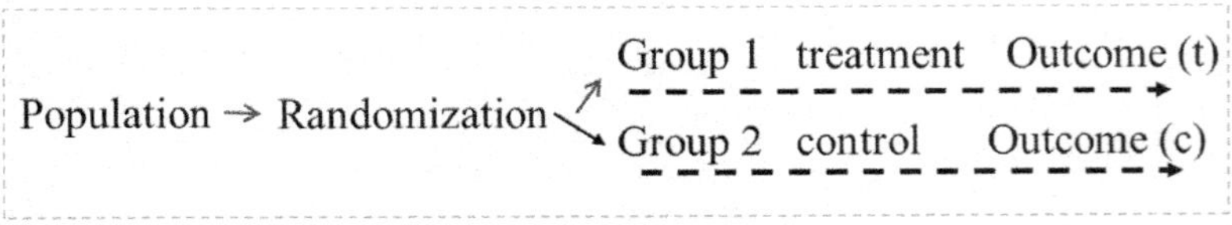

The flowchart shows two randomly assigned groups: the treatment and control groups. Neither of the two groups has been pretested. Posttest observations are carried out on both groups to assess the effect of the manipulation. Statistical analysis is used for two sample differences. A T-test can be used if the data is normally distributed.

Advantage: Random sampling sets the two groups equally, avoiding selection bias with a sufficient sample size; therefore, the outcome differences are due to intervention but not baseline variations. Pretest measurement could lead the participants to modify their responses, affecting the results. If we make two groups equal at the baseline by measuring pretest data, we lose random sampling, introducing selection bias. On the other hand, the baseline data may affect the researcher's random allocation of participants.

Disadvantage: The disadvantage is attrition bias is high due to possible high dropout rates for whatever reasons; therefore, this design is only suitable for short-term study. Moreover, there is no pretest data to compare when the outcome shows different responses, which is a significant drawback. Finally, the experiment requires a large sample size because of random sampling, making the project difficult to do.

A Pretest-Posttest Design

A pretest-posttest study has one placebo group and one intervention group. Researchers measure the baseline data or dependent variables before and after the intervention (pretest and posttest measures). Because this is a randomized controlled trial, researchers randomly allocate the participants into the placebo or intervention groups.

The procedures are as follows:

- Randomly assign participants to the intervention group and placebo group.
- Measure pretest data in both above groups.
- Apply the treatment or placebo.
- Examine the differences between the intervention and placebo groups.

Example: A researcher hypothesizes that a new exercise protocol promotes body flexibility. In this case, you may measure the baseline of body flexibility as pretest data and then measure the flexibility as outcome data after applying the exercise protocol as posttest outcomes. (See below figure, T: treatment; C: control).

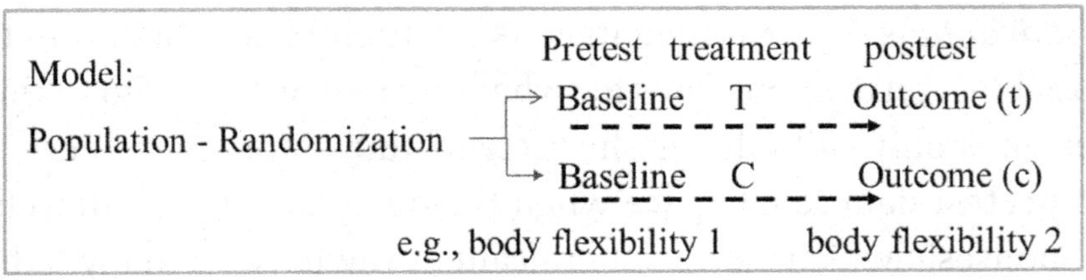

The above figure shows a mix of between-group and within-group design. Here, *between* means between the placebo and treatment groups. *Within* implies pretest and posttest measures within the same group. You could use a two-way repeated measure ANOVA for a possible treatment and time interaction effect since the same group was measured before and after the treatment.

You may see an example in a paper published previously (Dimitrov and Rumrill, 2003).

In addition, it is common to perform a pretest and posttest design without randomization or a single or double blind of subject allocation. For example, it would be challenging to do a randomized trial when you want to do a clinical study using inpatients and a small sample size. In this case, the study is a quasi-pretest-posttest study design; therefore, you may need to monitor the internal validity to reduce possible bias and confoundings.

Crossover Design

A crossover study is a longitudinal study containing two groups. They are the control and treatment groups. As an RCT, the researchers randomly allocate the participants into either a control or treatment group.

A crossover design is a robust research design to detect the treatment effect. You can use this design to conduct clinical research, dietary intervention, or exercise study. Since it is a within-subject design, the advantages are an equal distribution of characteristics, reduced data variation, and subjects exposed to more than one treatment as self-control. For example, a self-controlled case-control study performs an intra-individual comparison, meaning each case acts as its control. The outcomes are analyzed when the subjects are either exposed or not exposed to the risk factor. (See figure below.)

Given these advantages, you may consider a crossover design. However, a disadvantage is that if the first treatment has permanent learning effects on the second treatment, you should avoid an application of a cross-over design, which can affect the results of the outcome variables.

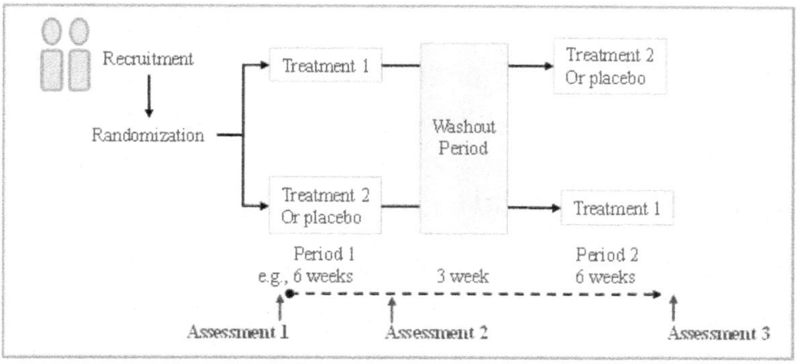

The figure shows that the pattern is the Group A and Group B to Group B and Group A study (a crossover design). Participants assigned to the Group A study receive treatment A first, followed by treatment B, and vice versa in Group B.

Advantages of a Crossover Design Are as Follows:

- An equal distribution of characteristics between the first and second treatments reduces the data variations.

- There is a reduced influence by confounding factors because patients act as their controls.
- A smaller sample size is required, as there is self-control.
- Patients will receive both treatments, making the project more attractive.

Disadvantages of a Crossover Design Are as Follows

- The first condition may influence the response to the second condition (i.e., carry-out effect). In this case, a crossover study should not be used.

An Extended-Level Design

An *extended level design* is suitable for the project requiring a large-scale study and dealing with complex questions. This type of design may require multiple research groups, multiple measurements, and a flexible or changeable platform.

A Simple Multi-Arm Trial

A *simple multi-arm* trial is also called an *umbrella trial*. It is that a single disease has several treatment groups. Here, several treatment groups share one control group. Researchers can evaluate multiple targeted therapies in several groups for a single disease (see figure below).

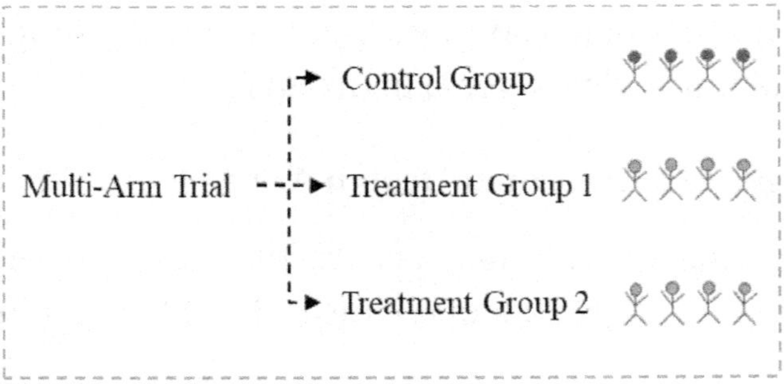

The advantage is that an increased number of treatment groups maximizes the chance of beneficial outcomes, thus making the study more likely to yield sufficient data to improve patient outcomes.

Example 1: Difference between subject groups: Genetic variation can lead to different responses to the intervention between participants. In this case, you can have multiple groups based on gene variations. Similarly, aging can lead to varying responses to the intervention; therefore, you can have multiple groups based on age (e.g., adolescent, young, and old). Similarly, such variations in participants can occur in response to the same diet, exercise protocol, or risk factors.

Example 2: Difference between the same category drug: You may use multiple groups of type 2 diabetic patients treated with metformin, gliclazide, and a placebo to control glucose levels. Another example is that researchers want to study the dose-response effects (e.g., low, medium, and high); therefore, you will need multiple groups.

All the above studies could use a simple multi-arm trial design.

A Basket Trial

A *basket trial* is a targeted intervention, meaning that the therapy has a single pathological target shared by several diseases. These diseases share some molecular changes or risk factors. Therefore, it is to perform a targeted treatment of multiple illnesses, sharing common pathological targets. For example, systemic inflammation occurs in chronic obesity, type 2 diabetes, and Alzheimer's disease. Anti-inflammation is the disease target for these diseases. Therefore, you may expect that anti-inflammation could benefit in alleviating the symptoms of obesity, type 2 diabetes, and Alzheimer's disease.

A Platform Trial

Rationale: A research area usually has several two-arm trials undertaken independently. As a result, it creates redundant and inconsistent control groups among the studies. Also, these separate two-arm trials can vary in research protocols or procedures. Therefore, the conclusion can be problematic, as the results are from heterogeneous studies (Park et al., 2021).

A platform trial is expected to have some standard protocols for a long-term study across multiple institutions. The same standardized procedures apply to all intervention and control groups. Researchers may include multiple interventions simultaneously. Commonly, these interventions share a control group and can have a pretest and several posttests, undergoing several interim evaluations.

The advantage of a platform trial is that the standardized procedures can harmonize the tests across different research groups to achieve comparable results. As a result, the study can generate an abundance of high-quality data. The design can make it possible to reduce patient numbers in the control group since the control group is shared among intervention trials. The design allows evaluating several treatments within the same clinical trial by spontaneously testing various drugs, protocols, or doses.

Furthermore, the structure of a platform trial is flexible, allowing new experimental arms to be added or the control arm to be updated if the standard control changes during the study.

Researchers can add a new treatment or stop a cure while the standard procedure does not need to be changed every time.

A platform trial may stop or replace a particular arm during the study. Since some trials investigating significant health issues can last for decades, some studies may need to be changed. For example, if an intervention does not work or has some errors, the researcher can remove that study or change to another study.

Also, platform trials can drop ineffective interventions and add new interventions during the trial while evaluating several interventions against a common control.

Follow-Up Trial

A *follow-up trial*, or *post-trial*, aims to monitor if the previous treatment has long-term effects on the disease or if any risk factors affect the progress. For example, the intervention effect may vanish after stopping the intervention for a certain period. Therefore, you may want to have a follow-up study. A follow-up study belongs to the cohort study, including exposure, time, and outcomes.

In many cases, a long-term follow-up study is vital for treatment efficacy and safety outcomes (Llewellyn-Bennett et al., 2016). This is because there are questions that patients, doctors, and families want answers to. In addition, some side effects and hazards may take a long time to emerge. An example of a follow-up study can be electronic health records published in a paper (Davies et al., 2018).

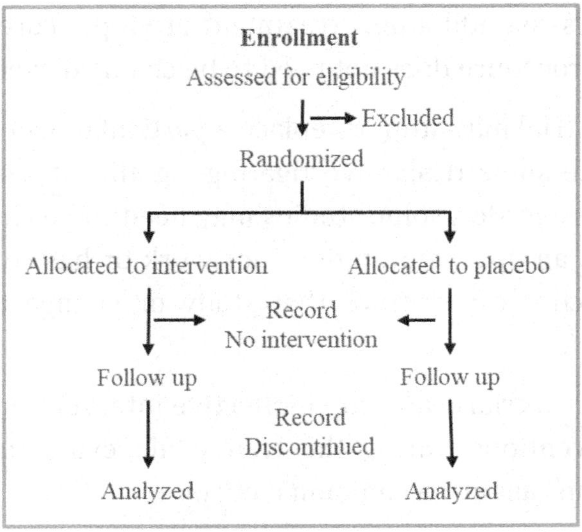

Examples of a Randomized Controlled Trial

Example 1: A RCT Uses a Linear Mixed Model to Investigate the Mean Difference

Although physical exercise benefits cognitive function, studies have shown some inconsistent outcomes in dementia patients. Therefore, researchers want to investigate the effect of exercise on cognition in dementia patients (Toots et al., 2017). Here, the design had the intervention and control groups with randomized subject allocation and a double-blind RCT design. The subjects were dementia patients. Using a repeated measure design, the researchers measured the baseline cognitive function as well as four and seven months after the exercise intervention. The researchers used MMSE and other tools to determine cognitive function. Having group and time factors, researchers examined the mean difference (95% CI, range, *p*-value) using linear mixed models.

Example 2: A Randomized, Double-Blind, Placebo-Controlled Trial Can Determine the Mean Difference and Time Effects

Rodent studies show that oligofructose supplements reduce obesity; however, such an effect has not been tested in human obesity. The researcher designed a randomized, double-blind, placebo-controlled trial that measured the body weight, composition, satiety hormone, food intake, and appetite ratings (Parnell and Reimer, 2009). A T-test determined Mean ± SD. The repeated-measures ANOVA with Bonferroni adjustment was for biochemical analysis. The meal test used an area under the curve to compare the intervention effects.

Quasi-Experiment Design

A *quasi-experimental design* covers a range of non-randomized interventions. Such research design is for when an RCT is unfeasible or presents ethical issues. For example, a researcher wants to investigate the effect of a new surgery protocol on patients before and after surgery, a follow-up study (Harris et al., 2006). However, the patients in this new protocol are of a small sample size, which does not allow randomization of patient allocation.

Causal or Non-Causal?

A quasi-experiment design will determine if the relationship between the variables is causal or not causal. For example, a well-designed quasi-study can address the cause-effect relationship between the intervention and outcomes. However, since it is not randomly sampled, the bias can be challenging to control. As a result, the cause-effect relationship may not be conclusive.

How Many Groups?

It depends on the aim of the study. A quasi-experiment can have only one group, for example, the muscle strength measured before and after interventions (pretest and posttest design). Or, the study can have two groups, one intervention group and one control group, but no random assignment of participants. It can also have multiple groups. Thus, it emphasizes an intervention targeting a population, but participants are not allocated randomly (Harris et al., 2004).

Qualitative and Quantitative Quasi-Experiments?

A quasi-experiment can be either *qualitative* or *quantitative*. Statistic methods used may vary from study to study. For instance, it can calculate the difference and association between two groups, develop a predictive value using regression analysis, or be a time-series design using repeated measure ANOVA.

Example: A researcher wants to test an exercise protocol to prevent falls by increasing leg muscle strength. The intervention is applied, and leg muscle strength is measured before and after the intervention. Here is a quantitative pretest and posttest quasi-experiment.

Types of typical quasi-experiments are as follows:

- Non-randomization is a feature.
- A parallel control group is not essential.
- Time-series study is common.

Strength of a Quasi-Experiment

A quasi-experiment can be used to investigate causality in a real-world setting without utilizing randomization and an equal-sized control group. This advantage makes it practical for clinical studies, such as a nursing study that only has a small sample size. Therefore, you may consider a quasi-experiment when a randomized controlled trial is not feasible because, for example, the sample size is small and/or there are ethical, personal, or location issues.

Weakness of a Quasi-Experiment?

There is no equivalence of controls and no randomization, which could introduce study bias and possible confounding factors.

A Quasi-Experimental Design with a One-Group Pretest-Posttest

In a quasi-experimental one-group pretest-posttest design, one group of participants is measured for the same dependent variable pretest and posttest interventions. The model features a pretest dependent variable (baseline dependent variable), intervention (treatment), and posttest dependent variable (outcome dependent variable) but no participant randomization of allocations.

	Dependent variable	Intervention	Dependent variable
No randomization	Baseline measure	Treatment	Outcome measure

The table shows a quasi-experimental one-group pretest-posttest design.

Data analysis: After the data is collected for baseline and outcome variables, normality and homogeneity tests are necessary to check the parametric test's suitability. A paired sample T-test will determine the differences between the baseline and outcome measures if the data is distributed normally. However, a Wilcoxon signed-rank test can calculate differences if the data is not distributed normally.

A Quasi-Experimental Two-Group Pretest-Posttest Design

A quasi-experimental two-group pretest-posttest design compares the changes between the two groups on the same dependent variable at the baseline and after an intervention, but with no randomization of participant allocations.

	Group	Dependent variable	Dependent variable
Non-randomization	Intervention	Baseline	Treatment
	Control	Baseline	Control

The table shows a quasi-experimental two-group pretest-posttest design. This mix of between- and within-group design requires a two-way repeated measure of ANOVA followed by post hoc analysis if the data is distributed normally. If the data is not distributed normally, you may apply a nonparametric analysis.

A Quasi-Experimental One-Way Repeated Measures Design

A quasi-experimental one-way repeated measures design focuses on time series. It aims to investigate the effects of treatment on participants over a defined period. It usually has a small sample size, and the interventions have the same group of participants. It is also called a *within-subjects design*. Sometimes, the baseline measure may not be possible.

DV	INV	DV	INV	DV	INV	DV
BL	T	O	T	O	T	O

The above table shows a quasi-experimental one-way repeated measure design. In this design, there is only one group of participants with the baseline and multiple outcome variables measured. Abbreviations: DV (dependent variable), BL (baseline), INV (intervention), T (treatment), O (outcome).

The features are (1) no controls, as each subject serves as its control; (2) the independent variables are the same. When the independent variable is the same, repeated measures analysis is used to analyze the variables; and (3) to test each independent variable separately.

Summary of Causal and Non-Causal Studies

A cause-effect study aims to identify the cause-and-effect relationship. So it is that a particular independent variable is a *reason* causing the outcome. The method is to use experimentation to establish a cause-and-effect relationship. Therefore, the event sequence is that the cause happened before the effect. The research design emphasizes the manipulation of independent variables in randomized controlled trials, well-designed cohort studies, or survey studies. You may need to measure outcome variables before and after an intervention. In a cause-effect analysis, avoiding potential bias and confounding factors is vital. Therefore, you need to carefully define independent, dependent, control, and confounding variables. An example of a cause-effect study can be that overeating high-fat food leads to increased blood cholesterol.

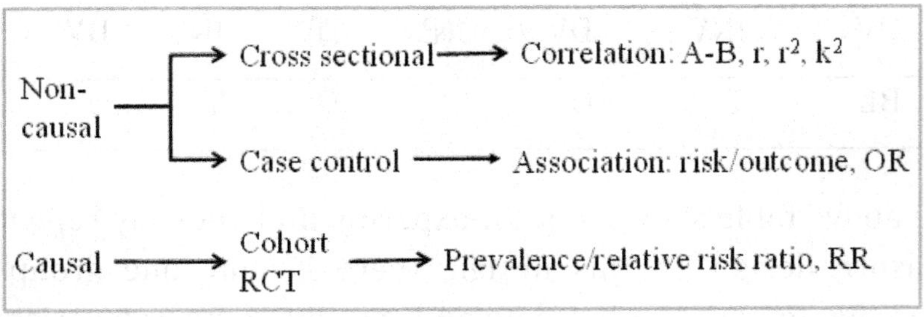

The above flowchart shows how the research design addresses the question of either non-causal (association only) or causal. The top panel shows the non-causal design studies. It includes a cross-sectional study and a case-control study. With a cross-sectional study, you may calculate a correlation coefficient r, coefficient of determination r^2, and coefficient of non-determination κ^2. In a case-control study, you can calculate all types of association values. The bottom panel shows the research designs addressing the causal effect, including a cohort study and randomized controlled trial.

A simple way to remember the meaning of *causal effect* is that B happened because of A, and B's outcome is strong or weak depending on how much, or how well, A worked.

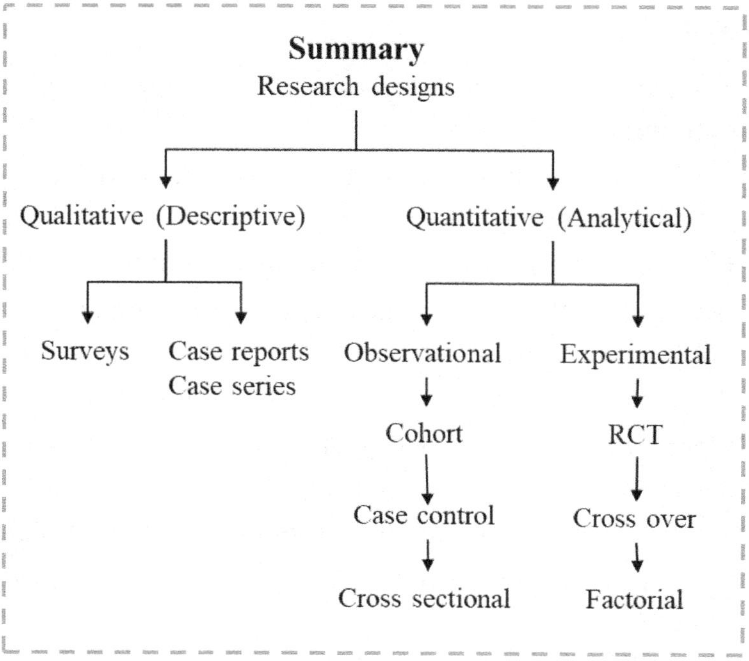

The above flowchart summarizes standard research designs.

ASK YOURSELF

- What is simple, block, stratified, and adaptive covariate randomization?
- What are the intention-to-treat analysis and the per-protocol analysis?
- What are the objectives of a randomized controlled trial?
- What are the advantages and disadvantages of a randomized controlled trial?
- Why is it preferred to use a double-blind design?
- What are the essential criteria for a true experimental design?
- What is a two-group random assignment posttest design?
- What is two-group random assignment pretest-posttest design?
- What are the advantage and disadvantages of a crossover design?
- What is the primary aim of a quasi-experimental design?
- What are the three types of quasi-experimental design?
- What are the strengths and weaknesses of quasi-experimental design?
- When do you use a quasi-experimental one-group pretest-posttest design?
- When should you use a quasi-experimental two-group pretest-posttest design?
- When should you use a quasi-experimental one-way repeated measures design?
- What are the essential procedures of the randomized controlled trial?
- How do you match the aim of the study and the type of research design?

CHAPTER 4

Sample Size and Statistic Power

TOPIC OUTLINE

- Alpha value
- Statistical power
- Effect size
- How to calculate effect size (Cohen's D)
- Control for random error
- Summary of sample size determination

Sample Size

The *sample size* is about statistically determining the number of samples required for a study. It is usually to estimate the minimum sample size needed for an experiment.

Samples are the number of observations taken from a population. It can be the subset of a region population, which can make an inference to the region. However, it should be representative. The larger the sample size, the more accurate the outcomes from an investigation.

Key Factors Affecting the Sample Size

Alpha Value

An *alpha value* is a probability of rejecting the null hypothesis assuming that the null hypothesis is true.

It depends on how sure you want to be of your answer, for example, 0.05 or 0.01. The sample size also depends on whether you consider the outcome one-sided or two-sided.

Example Alpha Value and H_0 and H_A Hypotheses:

H_0 hypothesis, if M1:M2:M3, $p > 0.05$, accept H_0, no further test is required; if M1:M2:M3, $p < 0.05$, reject H_0 or accept H_A. If you have three or more groups, it requires a post hoc analysis. Abbreviations: M = mean value, H_0, null hypothesis, H_A, alternative hypothesis.

Statistic Power

Statistic power is the probability that the test correctly rejects the null hypothesis when the alternative hypothesis is true. For example, if a study has 80% power, it means that the study has an 80% chance of the test having significant results. Most studies use 80% statistical power.

Effect Size

Effect size is the difference between the testing and control groups, or the size of the experimental effect.

What is your expected effect size for your study? Considering this question at the start of your research would be best. If the expectation is a large effect size, the relationship needs to be strong between the variables.

What are the acceptable bases used to determine the effect size?

- An estimate from pilot data
- An estimate from previous studies
- An educated guess

Calculation of the magnitude of effect:

- Formulation is % change = (M_2 – M_1) / M_1 x 100.
- For example, mean 1 = 16.5, mean 2 = 19.7
- The magnitude of effect is % change = (19.7 - 16.5) / 16.5 x 100 = 0.194 x 100 = 19.4%

Calculation of Effect Size

The effect size (ES) represents the standardized difference between two or more means. Here, we emphasize the standard deviation (SD).

$$ES = \frac{(M_{test} - M_{con})}{SD_{pooled} = \sqrt{(s_t^2 + s_c^2)/2}}$$

Calculate the ES of the treatment:	Calculate the ES of the treatment:
Group 1 test: Mean ± SD, 13 ± 3 Group 2 control: Mean ± SD, 9 ± 3	Mean 1 test = Mean 15.5, SD = 10.9 Mean 2 control = Mean 12.1, SD = 7.9
$= \frac{13 - 9}{\sqrt{(3^2 + 3^2)/2}}$ = 4/3= 1.33 (Cohen's d) This would be a large ES.	$= \frac{15.5 - 12.1}{\sqrt{(10.9^2 + 7.9^2)/2}}$ = 3.4/9.52= 0.36 (Cohen's d) This would be a small ES.

Cohen's D

Cohen's D indicates an effect size between treatment and control groups. It is the most commonly used to report the effect size in a T-test, ANOVA, and meta-analysis. Cohen's D is similar to Hedges's g. However, Hedges's g emphasizes the sample's SD while Cohen's D emphasizes the population's SD; however, they are not strictly used in the literature.

The magnitudes of Cohen's D:

- Cohen's D = 0 is no effect.

- Cohen's D = 0.2 is a small effect.
- Cohen's D = 0.5 is a moderate effect.
- Cohen's D = 0.8 or > is a large effect.

You can use ANOVA to calculate the effect size for the two groups; however, no effect size is provided if you use SPSS to do a T-test.

Example of manual calculation of the ES

- Group 1: Mean ± SD, 13 ± 3
- Group 2: Mean ± SD, 9 ± 3
- $= \frac{13 - 9}{\sqrt{(3^2 + 3^2)/2}} = 4/3 = 1.33$ (Cohen's d)
- This would be a large ES.

Online Calculation of Cohen's D

The below shows the method to calculate Cohen's D online, which requires the mean value and SD.

Example of online calculation of Cohen's *d* and the effect-size correlation, r_1, using means and standard deviations.

Website: https://www.uccs.edu/lbecker/

- Group 1: Mean ± SD, 13 ± 3
- Group 2: Mean ± SD, 9 ± 3

Cohen's d for effect size of difference between two groups.

Effect-size r for association explained between two groups.

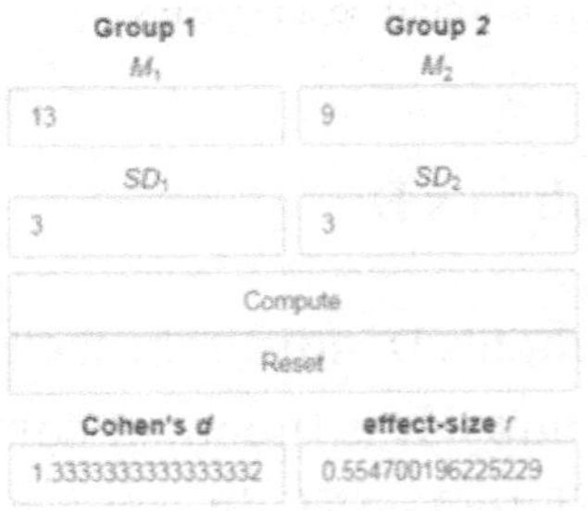

Use SPSS Software to Calculate the Effect Size

If there are more than two groups, you can use SPSS to calculate the effect size, which can be found as the partial eta squared value under "Univariate analysis of variance."

ES of a four-group study

Cohen's *f2* method of effect size is used to find out the effect size when you have more than two groups. This can be calculated for partial eta squared value.

- *Partial eta squared*
  - Report: F (3, 84)=20.183, p<0.000
  - Effect size: 41.9%

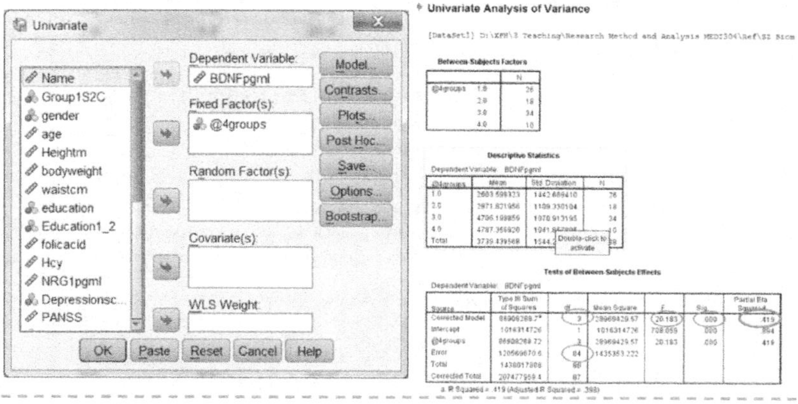

The above table shows an SPSS report about the effect size calculation.

Use a Shared Standard Deviation to Calculate the Sample Size

Here is an example: We want to work out the sample size for a new study (An et al., 2018). In this case, the mean value of the standard deviation was from a previous study. We used an online calculation. The website is http://stat.ubc.ca/~rollin/stats/ssize/n2.html. Note: You can manipulate the sample size to increase statistical power.

H. An et al. / Schizophrenia Research 192 (2018) 457–458

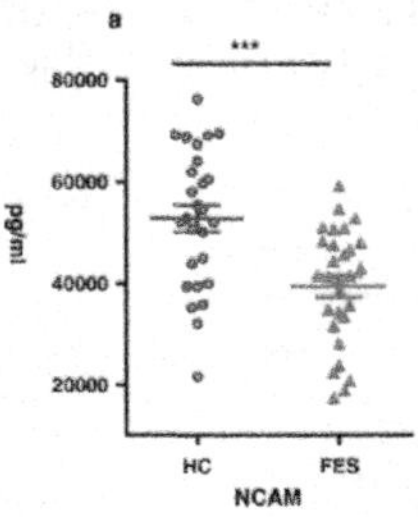

Fig. 1. The neural cell adhesion molecule (NCAM) concentration in the FES patients was 30% lower than normal controls. ***$p < 0.001$.

was a significantly positive correlation between the education and serum NCAM levels ($r = 0.362$, $p = 0.005$) considering all subjects.

Fig. 1 shows that the serum NCAM levels were 30% lower in FES patients compared with HC subjects (38.22 ± 12.99 μg/ml vs 54.82 ± 17.03 μg/ml, $p < 0.001$). Cognitive scores on MCCB were significantly lower in FES patients than healthy controls (87.00 ± 10.58 vs 56.67 ± 12.60, $p < 0.001$). The serum NCAM levels were positively correlated with the total scores of MCCB ($r = 0.438$, $p = 0.003$). Multiple regression analysis confirmed that serum NCAM level was an independent contributor to MCCB total Scores.

A doctor designs a project to study if plasma neural cell adhesion molecule (NCAM) is lower in patients with schizophrenia. How can he/she work out the sample size required for the project?

1. To find a previous work as reference.
2. Use the data: Mean 1, Mean 2 and common standard deviation; Calculate
3. Calculate power

- ◉ Calculate Sample Size (for specified Power)
- ○ Calculate Power (for specified Sample Size)

Enter a value for mu1: 38.22

Enter a value for mu2: 54.82

Enter a value for sigma: 15

- ○ 1 Sided Test
- ◉ 2 Sided Test

Enter a value for α (default is .05): .05

Enter a value for desired power (default is .80): 0.80

The sample size (for each sample separately) is: 13

Calculate

Use Population Data to Calculate the Sample Size

If the control group data from a previous study is unavailable, you can use population data to calculate the sample size. Here is an example from our earlier study. Patients with bipolar disorder often have an increased plasma uric acid level and a high prevalence of metabolic syndrome. We want to ask if hyperuricemia is associated with metabolic syndrome in these patients. To design a study, we need to work out the sample size. We found the below table from a previous study. It shows the patient data, but no control data was available. What do you do next? We found population data of our region, which has a 20% prevalence of metabolic syndrome. We then calculated the sample size or estimated (below). Although the estimated sample size is imperfect, this method provides the best estimation.

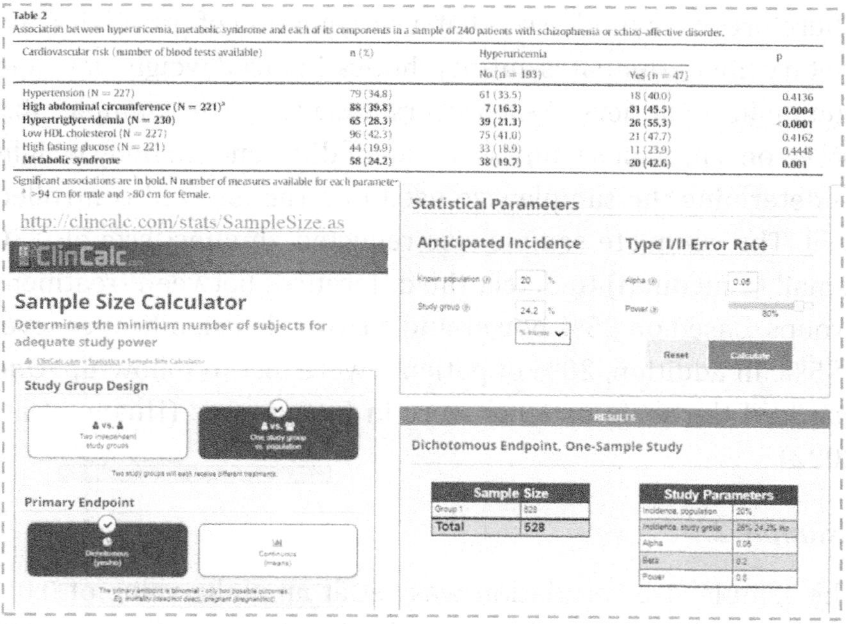

Table 2
Association between hyperuricemia, metabolic syndrome and each of its components in a sample of 240 patients with schizophrenia or schizo-affective disorder.

Cardiovascular risk (number of blood tests available)	n (%)	Hyperuricemia		p
		No (n = 193)	Yes (n = 47)	
Hypertension (N = 227)	79 (34.8)	61 (33.5)	18 (40.0)	0.4136
High abdominal circumference (N = 221)[a]	**88 (39.8)**	**7 (16.3)**	**81 (45.5)**	**0.0004**
Hypertriglyceridemia (N = 230)	**65 (28.3)**	**39 (21.3)**	**26 (55.3)**	**<0.0001**
Low HDL cholesterol (N = 227)	96 (42.3)	75 (41.0)	21 (47.7)	0.4162
High fasting glucose (N = 221)	44 (19.9)	33 (18.9)	11 (23.9)	0.4448
Metabolic syndrome	**58 (24.2)**	**38 (19.7)**	**20 (42.6)**	**0.001**

Significant associations are in bold. N number of measures available for each paramete
[a] >94 cm for male and >80 cm for female.

Description of the Sample Size in Methods

Here is an example: To ensure the study had adequate power, we calculated the required sample size based on a previous study of the mean 1, mean 2, and a common standard deviation. We had statistical power at 80% and a type I error level of 0.05 (alpha 0.05, two-tailed) or $p < 0.05$. And we had an effect size of 0.5 (or ranging from 1.4 to 2.0) with at least 80% power and a type I error level of 0.05 (alpha 0.05, two sided). Therefore, our sample size (345 cases and 396 controls) was deemed suitable for this study on the association between the variables.

Example 1: Sample Size in a Randomized Control Trial

Antipsychotic drugs can induce body weight gain leading to metabolic syndrome. However, probiotics and prebiotics (e.g., dietary fiber) effectively improve metabolic syndrome.

Therefore, we hypothesize that a combination of probiotics and dietary fiber attenuates antipsychotics-induced weight gain and metabolic disorders. Researchers calculated the sample size based on a previous study's treatment difference in body weight to determine the sample size used in a randomized controlled trial. The complete sample size reflected an effect size of 0.30 (small to medium) to detect the differences between treatment groups, based on 85% power and a two-sided significance level of 5%. In addition, 20% of patients were lost to follow-up. One hundred thirty-six patients were in four groups (Huang et al., 2022).

Example 2:

The sample size calculation was set at an alpha value of 0.05, power of 85% based on a previous study (ref). The possible confounding factors are marital status, illness duration, and episode numbers. All statistical tests were two-tailed, with the alpha level set at 0.05 (Chen et al., 2018).

Control for Random Error

Random error is an error occurring by chance. Usually, it is due to the sample size being too small. Small sample size is less likely to be representative. Generally speaking, an association study usually requires about three hundred samples.

A Random Error by Chance

For example, there are one hundred red balls and one hundred blue balls. If you put them together and randomly take two balls, it could be one red and one blue, two red but no blue, or two blue but no red. Therefore, the error is substantial to represent the red versus blue balls ratio. However, if you take one hundred balls, the chance of the error is reduced. If you take all balls, the ratio will be 50:50, representing the ratio correctly. Therefore, the smaller the sample size, the bigger the random error by chance.

Why are the results inconsistent for the same study reported in the literature? The inconsistency is mainly due to the sample size being too small for studies. When the sample size is too small, it generates a random error by chance. Consequently, the outcomes become inconsistent, e.g., higher or lower than the actual value.

For example, you may draw a conclusion based on multiple studies.

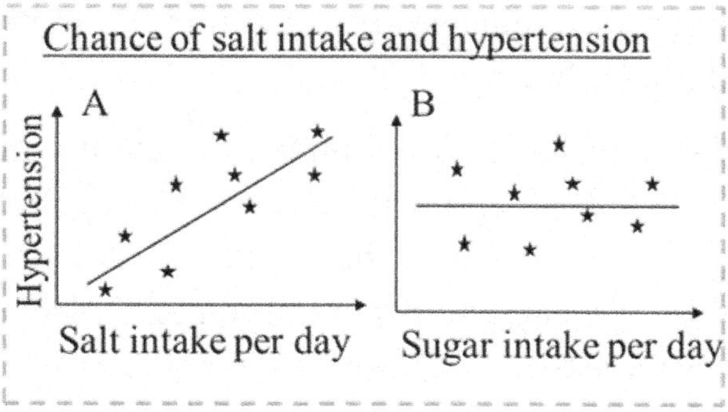

The above figure shows the analysis based on a review paper's data. Insert figures A and B, with nine stars, represent nine studies in each plot. Because these studies had small sample sizes, there are significant variations; however, the reviewer pulled the data together and created figures A and B. Figure A showed a positive correlation between high salt intake and hypertension; however, figure B showed no correlation between sugar intake and hypertension. These conclusions could not be drawn based on any single study.

Control for random error relies on the following:

- Sample size
- *p*-value
- Confidence interval

Sample Size Determination

The ideal sample size is determined by the alpha value, statistical power, and effect size.

In addition, the sample size also depends on the standard variations in the study population. The study will require a larger sample size if the sample has a large standard deviation. Standard deviation could refer to a similar or pilot study, general population, or your study population. The type of sampling (random) and type of analysis (e.g., the number of groups) can also affect the sample size.

What will be required for the sample size if you reduce the *p*-value from 0.05 to 0.01, and why? The answer is that the sample size needs to be increased because the statistical power contributes to the sample size requirement. Also, when the sample size is increased, confidence is increased.

The Magnitude of Effect

- Example: mean 1 =16.5, mean 2 = 19.7
- What will be the magnitude of the effect?
- % change = $(M_2 - M_1)/ M_1 \times 100$
- % change = (19.7 - 16.5) / 16.5 x 100 = 0.194 x 100 = 19.4%

The magnitude of the effect is 19.4%.

ASK YOURSELF

- What is an alpha value?
- What does it mean when a study has 80% power?
- How is the effect size calculated?
- What are the factors determining the sample size?
- What does a Cohen's D value of 0.5 mean?
- What is a random error, and how do you control it?

CHAPTER 5

Research Validity, Bias, and Confounders

TOPIC OUTLINE

- Internal validity
- External validity
- Enhance internal and external validity
- Selection bias
- Information bias
- Publication bias
- Halo effect
- Placebo effect
- Hawthorne effect
- Confounders

Internal validity

Internal validity is about our confidence in showing a difference due to the independent variable alone. It is a measure to ensure that a researcher's experimental design follows the cause-and-effect principle. It is about the cause-and-effect relationship. Internal validity aims to eliminate alternative factors for the outcomes rather than the outcomes being questionable. The higher the internal validity and the more confident we are in the results, the less chance the results are caused by confounding factors.

You could check the internal validity of whether or not:

- the cause leads to the effect,
- the cause and effect change spontaneously, and
- no other factors affect this relationship that you report.

Content Validity:

The test measures appropriate content. How accurately does a test or questionnaire measure the concept or evaluate the hypothesis? Content validity has face validity and logical validity.

Face Validity:

The test appears to test what it aims to test at face value. It is less rigorous than logic validity. For example, a test has a low face validity if you seek to test cognition and instead you measure depression. Since face validity is a subjective measure, it is often considered a weak form of validity.

Logic Validity:

The test involves a statistical approach and an expert who knows the topic to assess the content validity.

Construct Validity:

Construct validity is if a scale or test measures the *construct* (theoretical concept) adequately. The construct should match the specific measure or scale used in the research.

Example of Construct Validity

A doctor tests the efficacy of painkillers on chronic neck *pain.* The doctor asks the patients to rate their pain levels from one to ten. The subjective measures give the test construct validity since it measures the pain. That is, the test measures the construct from one to ten.

However, if the doctor instead measures depression, anxiety, and discomfort, the test has no or weak construct validity or wrong construct validity for measuring pain. Therefore, construct validity can help researchers check the research design.

Another example is that the construct validity for brain functions can include intelligence, ability, and emotion.

Threats to Internal Validity

Maturation:

Subjects change their status during the experiment. For example, children increase body weight and height over periods of growth. Another example is that the subject gets tired during the study. These factors can change the reaction to the intervention, which can happen during a chronic study.

Attrition:

Subjects drop out, which leaves the results with a biased sample, especially the control group. The bias is that participants do not choose to leave or are highly motivated subjects.

Background:

Events are not part of treatment. For example, researchers are studying exercise and health, but subjects do additional physical activity outside the study, which can threaten the internal validity.

Confounders:

Other variables associated with the treatment change the outcome.

Testing:

Learning and practice can affect the outcomes as confounders. The cause is due to repeated tests using the same measures. For example, if you had a person doing the same test three times, the person would learn the test. Therefore, the person is likely to do better the third time.

Instrumentation:

Changing instruments or tools can alter the outcomes. For example, the results may vary when recalibrating the instruments, changing the assessor, and changing the detection kit for biomarkers.

Statistics:

The analysis uses extreme scores or outliers, distorting the outputs. Or misuse of statistical methods between parametric and nonparametric analysis.

Selection biases:

The study uses non-random participant selection, meaning that groups are not equivalent.

Expectancy:

Researchers anticipate that certain subjects will perform better, influencing the analysis outcomes.

Controlling Threats to Internal Validity

Blinding: Participants do not know what treatment they receive.

Random allocation: Researchers randomly assign participants to treatment and control groups.

Control: Researchers design an appropriate control group to match the treatment group but only differ in the intervention.

Experimental manipulation: Researchers manipulate the independent variable instead of observing an association.

External Validity

External validity or *transferability* is about the generalization of research outcomes. *External* refers to how research findings can be generalized to other people, settings, times, measures, or actual practice. For example, randomized controlled trials need to consider external validity. In addition, external validity can help provide evidence to policymakers, public health researchers, and other researchers in their work.

Criterion validity:

Criterion validity describes how reliably one variable's measurement can predict another variable's response. The first is the explanatory variable, and the second is the criterion variable (see below figure).

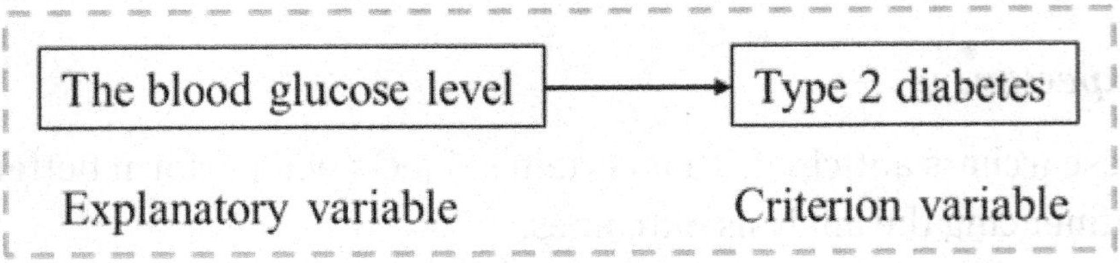

Example of Criterion Validity

The blood glucose levels may predict if the subject becomes diabetic in five years for the age range between fifty and sixty. You can use the Pearson correlation coefficient test to indicate the strength and direction of criterion validity. For example, suppose we collected data on blood glucose levels of two thousand subjects and recorded the subjects diagnosed with type 2 diabetes five years later. We found the correlation between the two variables was 0.8, highly correlated.

Criterion validity contains predictive validity and concurrent validity. In addition, criterion validity requires a standard for comparison, either a future or a current standard.

Predictive Validity:

The measurement of one variable can predict the measurement of the same variable in the future (future standard, see the above figure). For example, a test predicts later diabetic incidence on a related criterion: blood glucose levels.

Concurrent Validity:

Concurrent validity measures two variables simultaneously (concurrently) to examine if one variable is significantly associated with another. For example, concurrent validity can measure the outcome variable against a *benchmark* value, providing the same test. A high correlation indicates a strong criterion validity. For example, you can examine a new measurement against a standard (concurrent validity) for criterion validity.

Threats to External Validity

Specific Sampling:

Suppose you have investigated the biceps muscle strength among fifty year-two university students. In this case, your results can not represent the biceps muscle strength of all university students but only year-two university students.

Selection Bias:

A selection bias is an improper procedure for selecting the sample in a population. For example, you cannot use heart rate variability to represent the general population if you only studied heart rate variability in athletes.

Interactions:

External validity can be affected when there is an interaction between variables. It means that your results also rely on other variables (confounders).

Improving External Validity

Replication:

Researchers can conduct the study again with different samples or in other settings to see if they get the same results. Meta-analysis examines multiple studies to determine if an independent variable's effect is reliable, seen as the equivalent of replication. Therefore, you can use a meta-analysis or systematic review to evaluate the external validity of the results.

Inclusion and Exclusion Criteria:

Researchers should set up explicit inclusion and exclusion criteria because it helps to define the sample or population they study. Also, the included participants should represent the general population and reflect its geographic features.

Representative Sample:

The subjects included should match and be able to address the research question. The representative sample must be clear and precisely defined. For example, if a study is on cognitive decline in aging, the sample age needs to be defined and be even between the groups. If the survey is about depression in schizophrenia, the survey should not include depression patients with other mental illnesses.

Enhance Internal and External Validity

You may consider both internal and external validities when you design a study.

For example, a research project has good internal validity but is not relevant to the population; therefore, it is not high-impact research. It would be better to consider the outcome applications instead of rushing through the experimental design or only focusing on finding differences.

Conversely, you may conduct field research that is highly relevant to the actual people but doesn't have a reliable reason to cause the outcomes; therefore, the project also does not have a high impact.

Certain factors can enhance the internal and external validities, including the following:

- Sample randomization
- Appropriate control group

- Limiting extraneous variables (inclusion/exclusion criteria)
- Having adequate sample size, characteristics, and geographic representations of the population

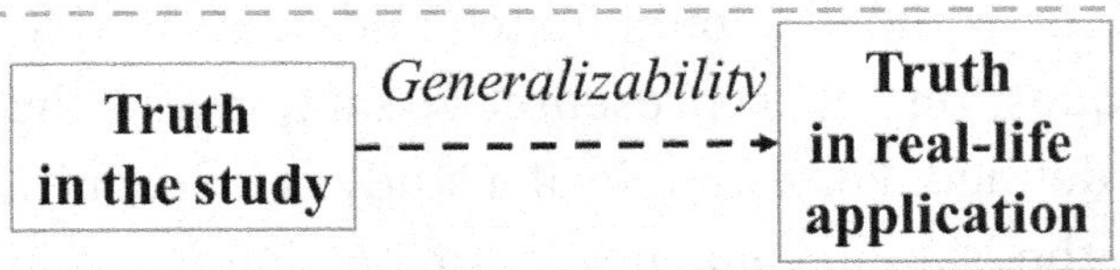

Internal validity	External validity
Produce solid results	Generalize findings
No outside variables	Real life application
Cause-effect relation	Population application
Best method accuracy	Translate to others

The above table shows the essential points of the internal and external validities for the experimental design. In summary, the project can reach a high impact and generate significant conclusions only if internal and external validities are high.

Bias

Bias is a process where the researcher or participant influences the results, which portray actual outcomes. Bias can lead to type I or type II errors.

Selection Bias

Allocation bias: Allocation bias belongs to selection bias. Here, the researcher allocates participants to groups based on their willingness, leading to differences in baseline characteristics between groups.

Self-selection bias: Participants select which group they want to join, which is a selection bias.

Inclusion and exclusion criteria bias: The researcher can consciously or consciously introduce bias, affecting a study's outcomes.

Addressing the above biases, researchers may use randomized allocation of participants.

Recruitment Bias

Sampling bias: This occurs when the researcher does not select the participants properly. For example, the researcher studies respiratory disease in an urban area without considering that people with chronic lung disease tend to move out of urban areas. It includes other biases, like migration bias or ethnic group bias.

Regional bias: This refers to a particular area differing from others. For example, those with psychiatric problems seek the anonymity of a city. Other examples include a place with limited English speakers who cannot understand the research questions or a region with a high aging population that cannot follow the research protocols. A regional bias should be avoided and precisely defined.

Dropouts

High dropout rates: Those who drop out of a study tend to differ from those continuing on the project.

Information Bias

Measurement bias: Assessment bias occurs if assessments lack objectivity. For example, subjective outcome measures are prone to exaggerate the effect.

Response bias: Participants provide inaccurate responses.

Observer bias: Observer leans toward some expected outcomes. The solution is to have blinding of assessors.

Publication Bias

Positive rather than negative results:

Some scientists publish results that trend toward the preferred results, usually positive ones. So it is because positive results are more likely to be accepted for publication; however, this can cause publication bias. A funnel plot of meta-analysis can indicate where the possible publication bias may lie.

Citation bias: Positive finding attracts more citations than negative findings. High-impact journal articles attract more citations than low-impact journal articles. We advise reading all relevant papers, or at least the ones from the last ten years, and then deciding which papers should be cited, leading to correct citations.

Outcome reporting bias: Selective reporting of some outcomes can occur, which can cause reporting bias. We should publish the results irrespective of whether the findings are positive, negative, or no change.

Halo Effect

Observer effect: The halo effect is observer-introduced cognitive bias. It relates to the observer's feelings, which are a bias. It belongs to the cognitive bias that influences the researcher.

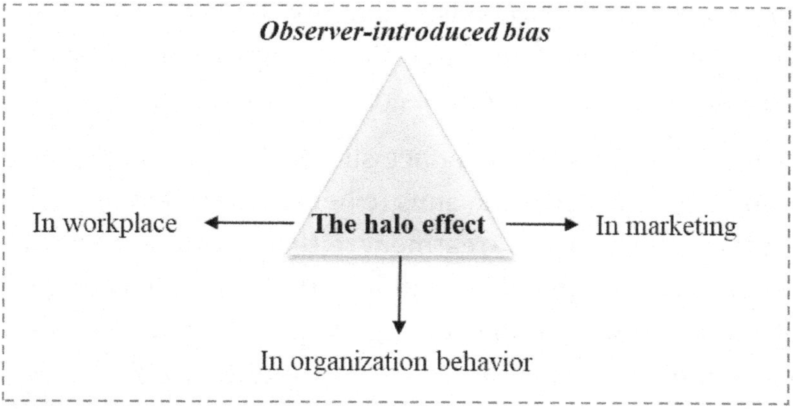

The above figure shows the halo effect, which the observer introduces bias. Observers' opinions can influence in many areas, such as external validity, internal validity and organizational behavior, and workplace performance.

Expectation effect: The researcher has expectations about a study. Using that feeling, the researcher assesses the experimental variables. It could refer to the tendency to judge a person or thing based on positive impressions from another area. For example, a researcher may appraise John's performance in swimming better than it is due to a positive first impression of his running speed.

Encouragement effect: This bias can give subjects more encouragement, influencing the results.

You can use multiple assessors or a double-blinded research design to reduce the halo effect.

Placebo Effect

Participants: The placebo effect is some participants' "known-expectation effect." It is the phenomenon by which participants experience a mental or physical effect after having a placebo or sham treatment. A placebo is a "dummy" treatment designed to have no known treatment value. For example, a placebo can be a sugar pill or capsule, water injection, or sham surgery.

Outcomes: The treatment effect should be different from the placebo effect. The placebo aims to help researchers understand the actual effect of the treatment, either positive or negative. However, the placebo effect can be a therapy for treating some health issues. For example, taking the placebo may help reduce anxiety in those who suffer from it. In addition, a placebo effect may trigger some hormone releases.

Existing drug or no drug: Today, in a clinical trial, it is preferred to compare a new intervention to an existing or old drug rather than an inactive placebo or no-drug pill. Do you know why?

Control: The characteristics of the placebo should be similar to the testing drug to minimize the participants' expectations.

Hawthorne Effect

Observer and participants: A *Hawthorne effect* combines the observer and participant effect. The original study was in the Hawthorne plant of the Western Electric Company in Chicago. When the manager increased the brightness, productivity increased due to the attention received under observation.

Outcome: The participant alters their behavior in response to the consequent awareness of being studied (McCambridge et al., 2014).

Control: How to control the Hawthorne effect? (1) hidden observation, (2) placebo, (3) appropriate control group, (4) multiple approaches.

Example of a Placebo-Controlled Clinical Trial:

The carers enrolled the patients in a follow-up trial after surgery, where carers monitored their recovery situations. After the surgery, the carers divided the patients into two groups, receiving minimal (group one) or intensive (group two) follow-up for six months. The minimal follow-up received an abbreviated baseline assessment and final cognition assessment; however, the intensive follow-up had a comprehensive baseline assessment and four behavioral assessments. The outcome showed that the patients achieved better results in response to the intensive follow-up than those on the minimal follow-up. Therefore, the Hawthorne effect under intensive follow-up has a better patient outcome due to patients' intensive attention.

You may find the following paper that reported a placebo-controlled clinical trial. The title of this paper is "The Hawthorne Effect: a Randomized Controlled Trial" (McCarney et al., 2007).

Confounders

Confounders are often known as the variables that correlate with the dependent and independent variables (Pourhoseingholi et al., 2012). A confounder is associated with both an outcome and a risk factor, making the two seem causally related. Therefore, it can lead to an incorrect explanation of the result.

Confounders or confounding variables are the variables possibly competing with the independent variable of interest. That is a problem because one feature of study subjects is not separated from another feature. A confounder is not a causal factor between exposure and consequence.

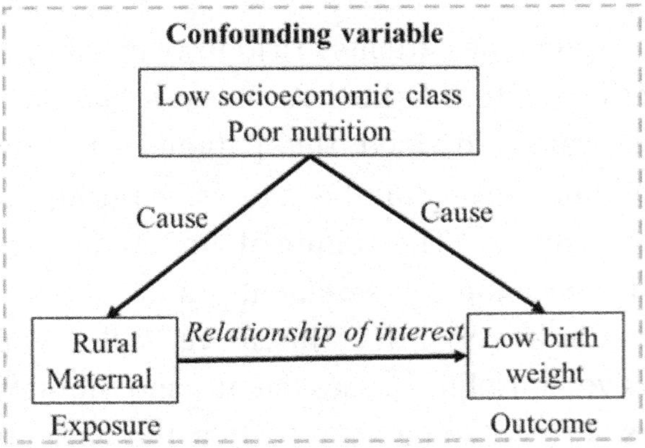

The figure shows an example of a confounding variable. The researcher concludes that there was a relationship or correlation between rural maternity and low birth weight, which could be incorrect. This relationship may be somewhat due to confounding factors such as low socioeconomic class and poor nutrition indicated in the figure above. Therefore, without an appropriate control for confounders, one cannot conclude that the low birth weight is due to rural maternity.

A confounder is not the causal factor between exposure and consequence. Common confounding factors of human studies are age, income, gender, and ethnic background.

A Better Understanding Of A Confounding Factor

A confounder is as follows:
1. Associated with exposure and often exists before exposure
2. Associated with the outcome
3. Not caused by exposure

Example 1: Causal Map:

A causal map emphasizes that *time* is critical in evaluating whether or not the factor is a confounder.

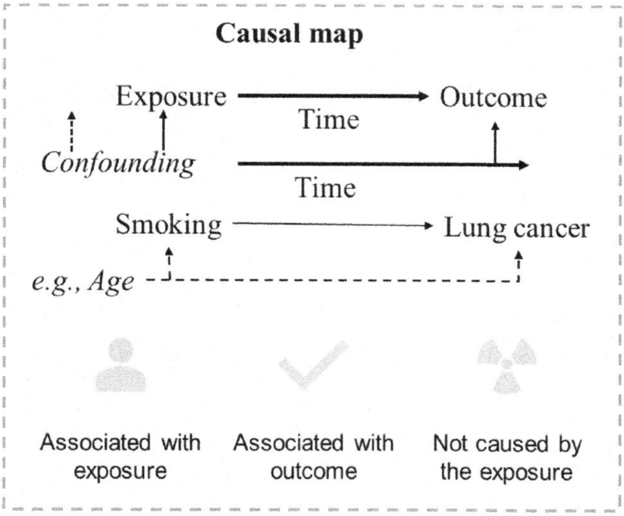

The above figure shows an example of a causal map. Smoking causing lung cancer does not happen in days or weeks. The exposure can take months to years to cause an outcome. A confounder (e.g., age) may accompany the causal factor for the entire course of disease development; however, confounders always occur before exposure. In this case, age (young or old) is associated with smoking and lung cancer, but age does not cause cancer. Therefore, age is a confounding factor.

Example 2:

Researchers found that people who carry matches likely develop lung cancer. Also, smoking is associated with people carrying matches and having lung cancer. However, carrying the matches does not necessarily cause smoking. Maybe there are other reasons people carry a box of matches around. Therefore, the conclusion (first sentence) is wrong, although it is a fact.

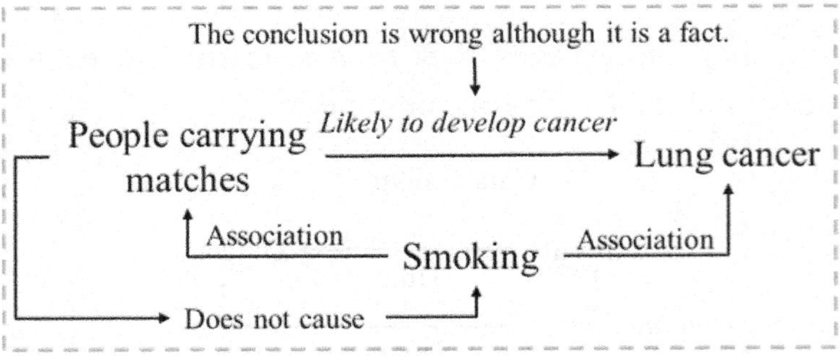

Example 3:

Researchers found that people drinking alcohol are likely to develop heart disease. Smoking is associated with alcohol intake and heart disease; however, alcohol intake does not necessarily cause smoking. Therefore, smoking is a confounder.

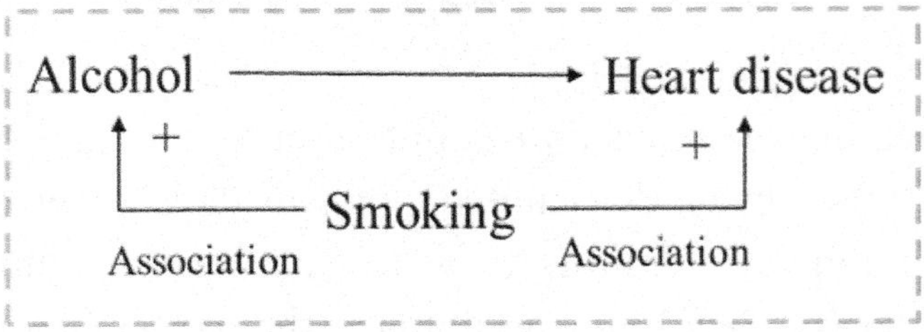

Example 4:

Researchers found that physical activity reduces myocardial infarction. Also, young age is positively associated with physical activity but negatively associated with myocardial infarction; however, physical activity does not cause young age. Therefore, young age is a confounder.

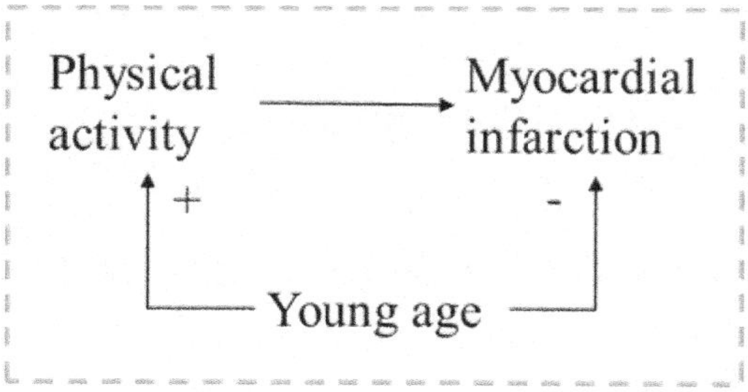

Example 5:

Researchers found that physical activity reduces myocardial infarction. Also, water intake is associated with physical activity: if people do more exercise, they will drink more water. However, water intake is not related to myocardial infarction. Thus, water intake is not a confounder.

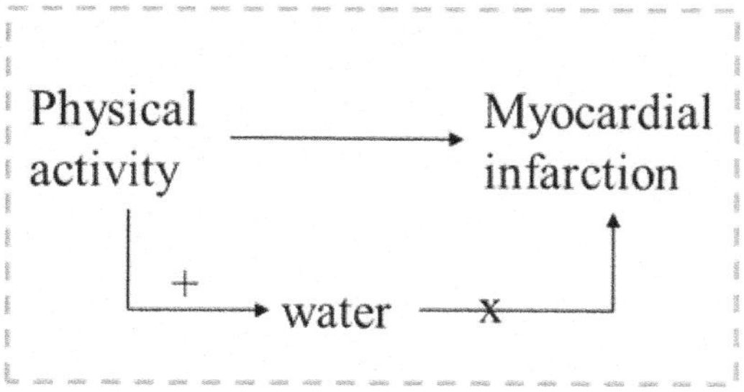

Example 6:

Researchers found that physical activity reduces myocardial infarction. Also, blood pressure is positively associated with myocardial infarction and negatively related to physical activity.

High blood pressure increases the chance of having a myocardial infarction. However, physical activity *does cause* blood pressure to decrease. Therefore, blood pressure is not a confounder.

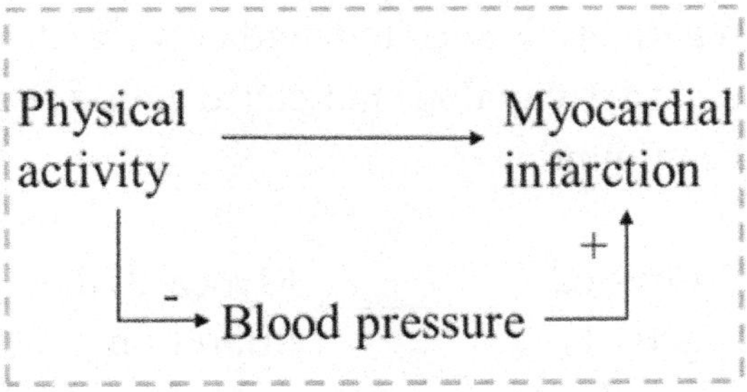

Do you know what the fundamental differences between bias and confounding are?

Bias creates an association that is *not true.* Confounding describes an association that *is true* but potentially misleading.

ASK YOURSELF

- What is the definition of *internal validity*?
- What is the meaning of content, face, logic, and construct validities?
- What are the possible contributing factors that threaten internal validity?
- How do you control for the threats to internal validity?
- What is the definition of *external validity*?
- What are the factors threatening external validity?
- How do you improve the external validity of your research?
- What is the definition of *bias*?
- What are the main types of selection bias?
- What are the main types of information bias?
- What is the halo effect? Why can it affect internal validity?
- What is a placebo effect?
- How do you control the Hawthorne effect?
- What are the criterion, concurrent, and predictive validities?
- What are the three critical criteria for confounders?
- What is a *causal map* used to evaluate whether or not the factor is a confounder?
- What are the fundamental differences between bias and confounders?

PART TWO

Data Analysis

CHAPTER 6

Data Type and Distribution

TOPIC OUTLINE

- Terminology of the data
- Data types
- Measurement scales
- Bell-shaped distribution
- Skewness
- Kurtosis
- Normality test
- Q-Q plot
- Box plot
- Homogeneity of variance
- Central tendency

Data Types

Data are the values you measure or record in your study. Two types of data are quantitative data representing amounts and categorical data representing groups.

Data: Data is information. It consists of individual numbers or measurements collected and organized for analysis.

Population: A population is a complete set of individuals, an all-inclusive group. In medical research, a population is a large pool of participants for a study.

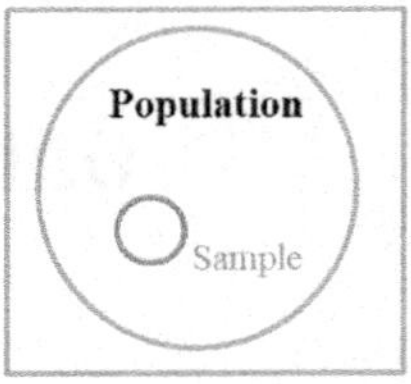

Sample: A sample is a subset of a population, as indicated below.

Biostatistics: Biostatistics is the application of biological data collection and analysis for biology, health, and medicine. Biostatistics also helps the design of biomedical, medical, and health experiments.

Quantitative data: The quantitative data is discrete or continuous numerically. Discrete variables count individuals, such as the number of students and chairs. Continuous variables measure nonfinite values, such as weight, blood glucose levels, and age.

Qualitative data: Qualitative data is about the quality of things. For example, there are ten observations.

Categorical data: Categorical data is information representing variables by class or categories, such as gender.

Time series data: Time series data is arranged in chronological order.

Categorical variable: The categorical variable is also called *nominal variable* or *discrete variable* with the information in categories, such as age and gender.

Numerical variable: The numerical variable is the variable in numbers.

Measurement Scales

The measurement scales in statistics include nominal, ordinal, interval, and ratio data.

Nominal Data

The *nominal data* is the "name" or variables without any quantitative values.

Examples:

- What is the patient's sex?
- Male and female (dichotomous)
- What is the person's hair color? Brown, black, blonde, gray
- Where do you live? NSW, SA, WA
- A person's name

Ordinal Data

The *ordinal data* can be rank ordered. It is the order of the values' significance, but their differences are unknown.

Examples:

- How do you feel? Very happy, happy, fine, unhappy, very unhappy
- How satisfied are you with our service? Very satisfied, satisfied, unsatisfied, very unsatisfied
- Education years: 1 = less than high school; 2 = high school degree; 3 = college degree; 4 = HDR degree.

Interval Data

Interval data is a numeric scale. The increments are consistent and measurable. There are exact differences between the values.

Examples: Celsius temperature, body weight gain

Ratio Scale

The ratio scale is an interval scale concerning a rational zero. It is the exact value for descriptive and inferential statistics. Since the 0 in the ratio scale means the complete absence of anything, there are no negative numbers on this scale.

Examples:

- Age. The clock starts ticking when you are born, but the age of zero technically means you do not exist. Also, there is no negative value.
- Weight. You would weigh nothing at 0 kilograms and, therefore, not exist.
- Height. If you were 0 centimeters, you would have no height.

Table. Summary of data types and scale measures

	Nominal	Ordinal	Interval	Ratio
The order of value is known		+	+	+
Frequency of distribution	+	+	+	+
Mode	+	+	+	+
Median		+	+	+
Mean			+	+
Quantifiable			+	+
Can add or subtract			+	+
Can multiple or divide			+	+
Has true zero			+	

Summary

In all four data types, nominal is only "name" data, whereas ordinal, interval, and ratio data have values. All four data types can use frequency and mode to show their values. The median value is for the data types where an order of the values is known. The mean is for both interval and ratio data. Both interval and ratio data can be quantified, added, subtracted, multiplied, and divided. Interval data is the only type of data that has a true zero.

Data Sampling

Data sampling is the selection of a subset of individuals from a large population. Sampling aims to establish a hypothesis concerning the characteristics of a population.

When designing a new study or analyzing existing data, how might you perform data sampling?

1) Define the population,
2) Determine the characteristics and location,

3) Determine the methods of probability sampling and non-probability sampling,
4) Determine sample size, and
5) Collect data.

Probability sampling: Probability sampling gives every member of a population an equal chance of being selected. This type of sample has the best chance of representing a population. Probability sampling includes random sampling and stratified sampling.

Random sampling: Random sampling involves:

1) Defining the sample, e.g., health, age, and gender;
2) Ensuring that each member of the population has an equal chance of being chosen;
3) Considering the location of the sampling;
4) Eliminating bias, e.g., setting up inclusion/exclusion criteria (potential bias);
5) Avoiding the selection of group location by subjects (selection bias); and
6) Using a table of random numbers or computer programs to randomize the sample.

Stratified sampling: Stratified sampling involves subdividing the population into strata or layers and randomly sampling each. This method is based on their similarities or common features. You will need to select representative subgroups, know the whole population's distribution percentage, and then use a similar distribution pattern in the sample group. This method will ensure that the subgroups are representative of the people. The advantage of stratified sampling is greater accuracy than other methods; therefore, a smaller sample size may be acceptable.

Table of stratified sampling

Population Age (Years)		**Sample Age (Years)**	
35 to 44	40%	35 to 44	40%
45 to 54	30%	45 to 54	30%
55 to 64	20%	55 to 64	20%
65 to 75	10%	65 to 75	10%

Non-probability sampling: Researchers must rely on available resources and sometimes can't perform probability sampling. In such cases, non-probability sampling is performed. Unlike probability sampling, non-probability sampling does not give every member of a population an equal chance of being selected. When data is collected from a simple accessible or available group, it is called convenience sampling or available sampling. The disadvantage of non-probability sampling is that this method is prone to bias, and the resulting sample may not represent the population, resulting in invalid external validity.

Bell-Shaped Distribution

A *bell-shaped distribution* is a common type of distribution for a variable. The data is distributed normally.

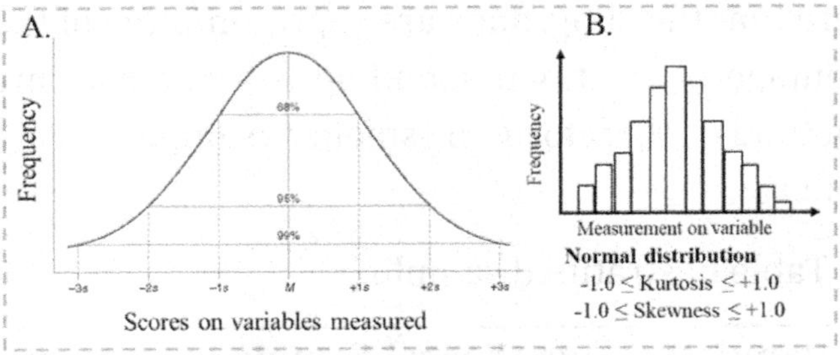

The above figure shows that the shape of the graph has a bell curve consisting of symmetrical data distribution (A). The data distribution is symmetrical, as it appears the same to the left and right of the center line. The width represents the standard deviations indicated in the figure (e.g., +1s, +2s). The mean (M) identifies the position of the center, and the standard deviation determines the width of the bell.

Figure A also shows that 68% of the data is within one standard deviation, 95% within two standard deviations, and 99% within three standard deviations from the mean.

Figure B shows a histogram with the data in a normal distribution. Here, the horizontal axis is the measurement of the variable of interest. The vertical axis is the probability of each outcome with corresponding points on the horizontal axis.

Skewness

Skewness measures the data's symmetry or lack of symmetry.

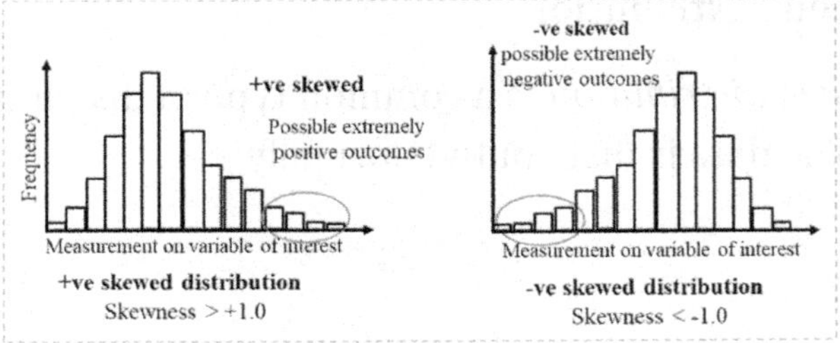

Skewness Indication

1) A normal distribution has skewness values ranging between –0.5 and +0.5.

2) Moderate positive skewness has skewness values between +0.5 and +1.0.

3) Extremely positive skewness has a skewness value of > + 1.0.

4) Moderate negative skewness has skewness values between -0.5 and -1.0.

5) Extremely negative skewness has a skewness value of < - 1.0.

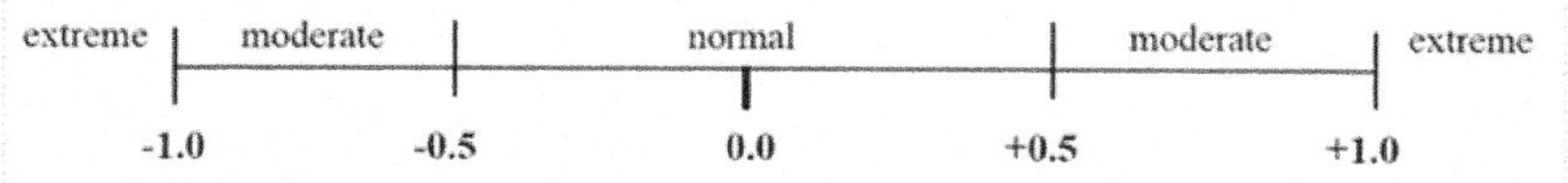

Data skewness indication

The below figure shows positive (A) and negative (B) skewed data. A positive skewness value (+1.60) indicates that the data is skewed to the left, whereas a negative skewness value (-1.60) indicates data is skewed to the right. This data is not distributed normally.

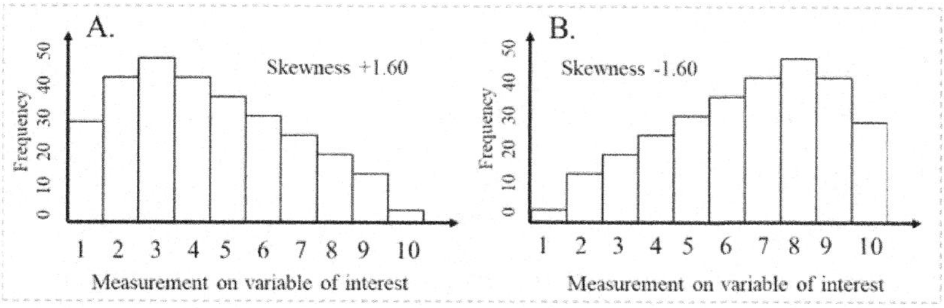

Kurtosis

Kurtosis indicates the distribution of event outcomes if a distribution is too peaked or too flat.

Statistically, kurtosis measures either tail's extreme values (left or right, see figure below). Excess kurtosis means the distribution of event outcomes has many instances of outlier results, causing fat tails on the bell-shaped distribution curve. Normal distributions have a kurtosis of three.

SPSS reports excess kurtosis, which is "kurtosis -3." Therefore, SPSS reports that a normal distribution has a kurtosis value of zero, meaning that SPSS calculates the excess kurtosis.

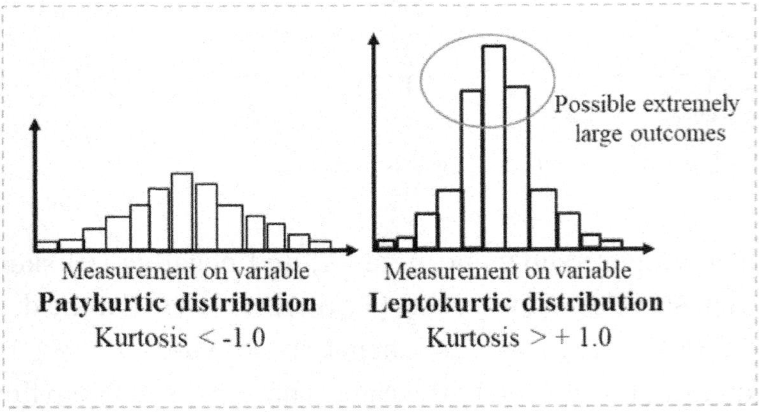

SPSS Kurtosis Report

- Data with a normal distribution has kurtosis values between -1.0 and +1.0, or mesokurtic.
- When the kurtosis value exceeds +1.0, the data is too peaked or leptokurtic. Therefore, there may be more extreme outliers than in a normal distribution in this case.

- When the kurtosis value is less than -1.0, the data is too flat or platykurtic. There may be fewer extreme outliers in this case than in a normal distribution.

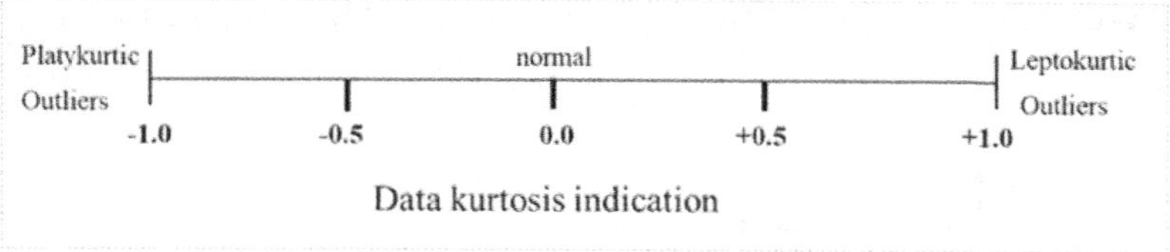

Response distribution: The figure below shows the distributions' characteristics between the dotted and solid lines. The data is symmetrical if a line is drawn through the middle of the solid line, which is also true for the dotted line. However, it demonstrates that although both curves are symmetrical, their shape can vary significantly. For example, the solid line has a much higher peak than the dotted line, even though both have a normal distribution.

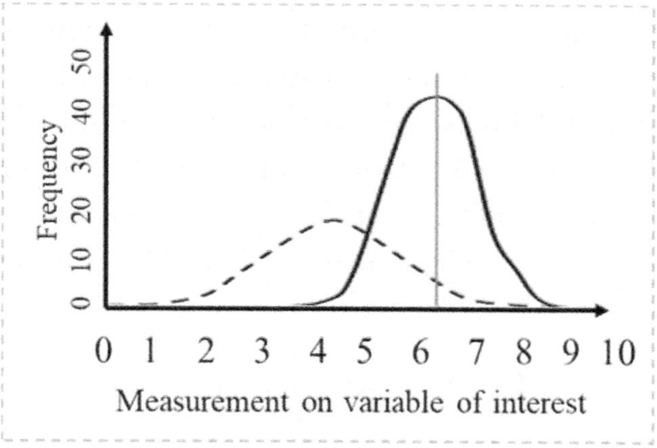

A bimodal distribution

A bimodal distribution has two peaks or modes. (See figure below.) The "mode" means the dataset's most frequent number or value. The bimodal distribution has one overall mode (the circle on the left is 60, the most frequent number) and a local mode (the circle on the right is 80). Bimodal data analysis should separate two modes instead of combining them. If you combine the two, the average value is about 70, which is misleading.

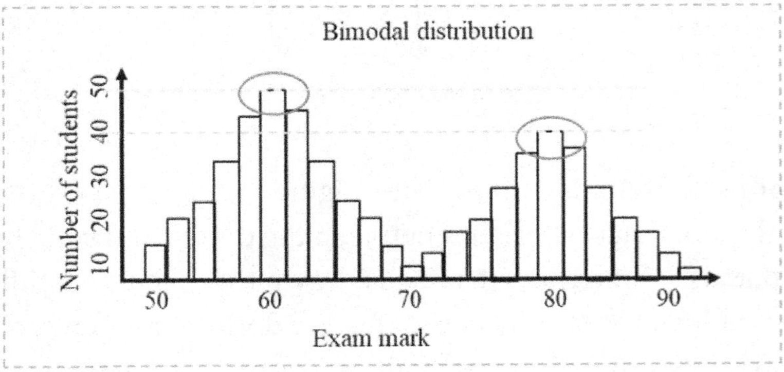

U-Shaped Distribution

Data with a *U-shaped distribution* is in a frequency or probability distribution shaped like the letter U. A U-shaped curve depicts a non-linear relationship between two variables. The U-shaped distribution has the maximum frequencies at both ends of the range of the variable. For example, a U-shaped distribution may occur in the number of people infected by the flu per year by age (see figure below). The highest frequency of flu is in young and old age groups.

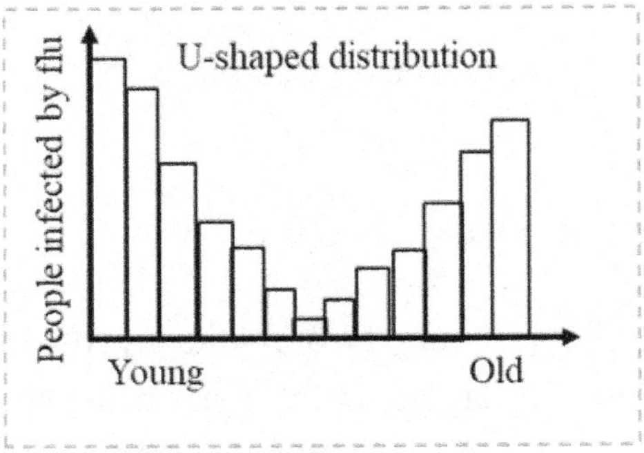

An inverted U-shaped distribution: The least frequent values are at both extremes, with the most frequent values in the middle of the distribution in an inverted U-shaped distribution.

When the doses are too low or too high, it can result in health risks in physiology; however, a moderate amount is expected to be beneficial in an inverted U-shaped distribution. For example, this is true for vitamin, exercise, triglyceride, cholesterol, pressure, and polyunsaturated fatty acid levels.

For example, vitamins are essential for life. A lack of vitamins causes adverse responses. However, excess vitamins can also cause adverse effects, thus giving rise to an inverted U-shaped dose-dependence curve.

Normality Test

The *normality test* determines whether sample data has a normal distribution. Generally, the Shapiro-Wilk test is thought of as being for sample sizes less than fifty, but it can be used on samples as large as two thousand. The Kolmogorov-Smirnov (K-S) test can be used for sample sizes larger than two thousand, is a more generalized analysis, and has low power.

The Shapiro-Wilk test is the most commonly used test for data normality. The value should not be significant to meet normality requirements.

The Kolmogorov-Smirnov test is used for a large sample size. When the outcome is insignificant, you may assume the data is in a normal distribution.

The table below illustrates the result of two alternate tests for normality using the SPSS computer software.

Tests of Normality

		Kolmogorov-Smirnov[a]			Shapiro-Wilk		
	Gender	Statistic	df	Sig.	Statistic	df	Sig.
Hightincm	male	.197	25	.013	.930	25	.086
	female	.187	24	.030	.925	24	.075

a. Lilliefors Significance Correction

On the right of the table: The Shapiro-Wilk test shows that the data of male and female heights have p-values of 0.086 and 0.075, respectively. Both p-values are greater than 0.05; therefore, both data have normal distributions. Because data have passed the normality test, further parametric analysis can be applied. Failure of the test for normality usually requires nonparametric analysis.

On the left of the table: The Kolmogorov-Smirnov test compares sample scores to a normally distributed set of scores with the same mean and standard deviation. The K-S test will determine if the two data sets differ significantly. Both males and females have p-values of less than 0.05. However, the sample sizes are too small (25 and 24) for the results of the K-S test to be used. We should therefore use the results of the Shapiro-Wilk test. A footnote shows that the K-S significance is Lilliefors corrected.

Q-Q plot

Q-Q plot stands for a *quantile-quantile plot*. This type of plot usually is used to determine whether or not a sample of data follows a normal distribution. Here, the Q-Q plot shows data distribution against the expected normal distribution. For example, the points will lie on a straight diagonal line as normally distributed data (A). However, if the plotted values vary from a straight line, the data is not distributed normally (B).

normally

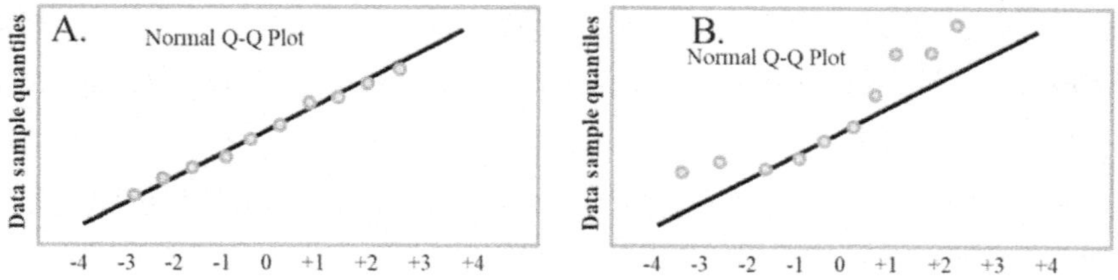

Histogram

The *histogram* indicates symmetrical, moderate-tailed distribution, which indicates that the data is in a normal distribution. The easy way to determine if data is distributed normally is to see if data is approximately bell shaped and symmetrical in a histogram. (See figure below.) When the histogram is not bell shaped, it suggests that the data is not normal.

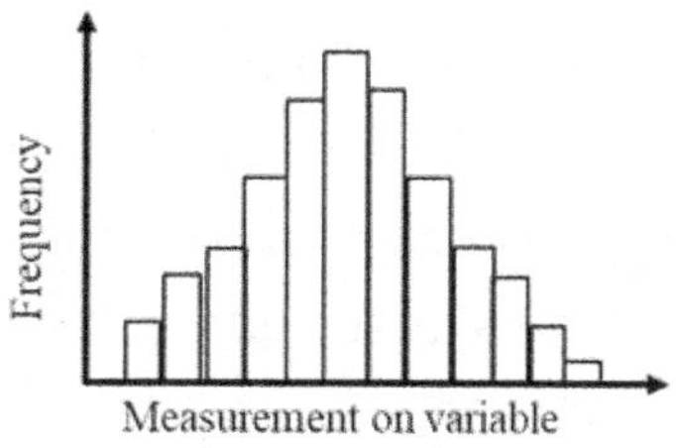

Q-Q plots and histograms give a quick visual evaluation of a normal distribution.

Box Plot

A *box plot* displays data distribution and depicts numerical data (skewed) groups via their quartiles. It shows the data set based on a five-number summary: *minimum, first quartile, median, third quartile*, and *maximum*.

A thick solid line corresponds to the median value. The median value is usually used in skewed data. This means that half of the values are lower than the median value and half of the values are higher than the median value. The first quartile line is the median value of the lower 50%, and the third quartile line is the median value of the upper 50% values.

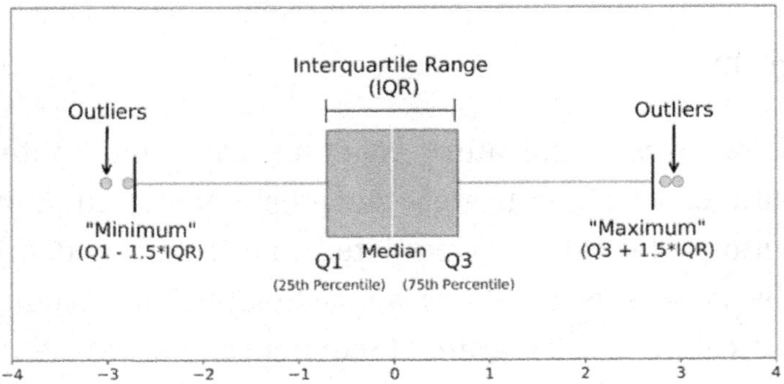

Homogeneity of Variance

If you want to compare data from different groups, the groups should have the same variance or homogeneity of variance. Levene's test is used to assess if the groups have equal variances. The outcome of Levene's test should not be significant if the groups have equal variances.

Levene's Test

A *Levene's test* assesses the equality of variances for a variable calculated for two or more groups. Levene's test assesses that the variances of the populations from which different samples are drawn are equal (null hypothesis).

When do you need to use Levene's test? It is used before a comparison of means. When Levene's test shows a significant difference, one should switch to more generalized tests, e.g., nonparametric tests.

The table below is a report of SPSS analysis showing group statistics, an independent samples test, and a Levene's test for equality of variance.

A SPSS Report

Independent Samples Test

		Levene's Test for Equality of Variances		t-test for Equality of Means					95% Confidence Interval of the Difference	
		F	Sig.	t	df	Sig. (2-tailed)	Mean Difference	Std. Error Difference	Lower	Upper
BMI	Equal variances assumed	9.925	003	5.327	47	000	3.308	621	2.059	4.557
	Equal variances not assumed			5.397	34.965	000	3.308	613	2.064	4.552

The table shows body mass index (BMI) statistics in patients with bipolar disorder and healthy controls. The table shows Levene's test values when comparing the data distribution between bipolar and control group data sets. In this example, $p = 0.003$; therefore, the null hypothesis of equal variances is rejected. It is concluded that there is a difference between the variances in the two populations. Therefore, the data should be considered for nonparametric analysis.

Central Tendency

A *central tendency* is a central value or a typical value for a probability distribution. A central tendency describes a data set using a single value located at the center of a data set.

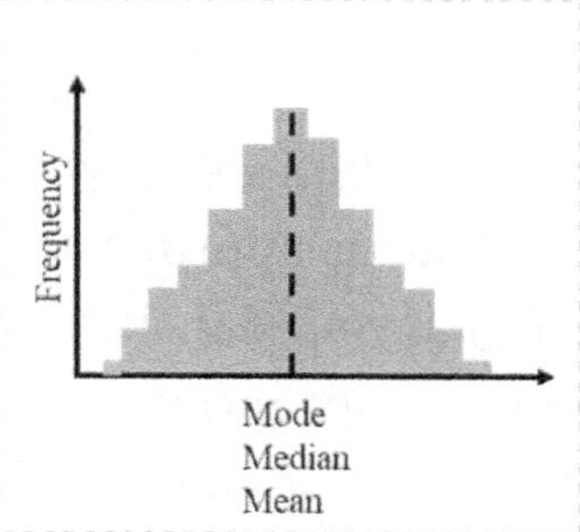

The main measures of central tendency are mean, median, and mode, which are used under different conditions. The figure shows that the mean, median, and mode are equal in a normally distributed data set.

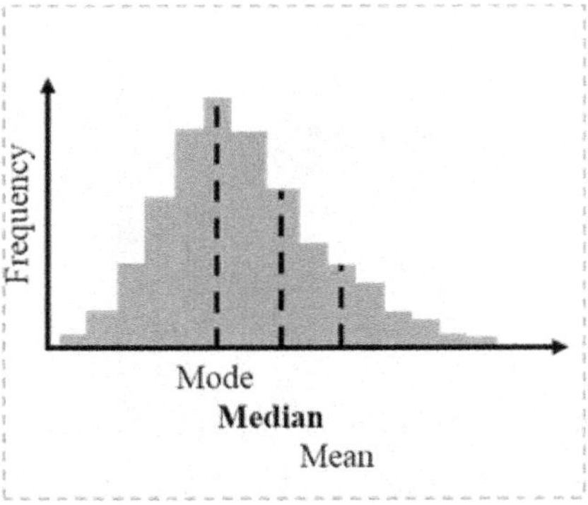

The figure shows that the mean, median, and mode have different values in data sets with a skewed distribution. It is noted that the median value is less affected by skewness compared to the mean and mode values. The mean is particularly sensitive to the influence of outliers.

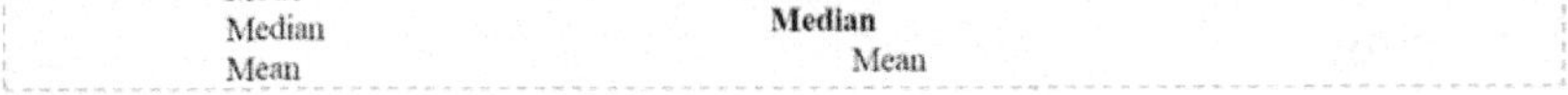

Which measure of central tendency should you use in your data set? This depends on your data set. If your data has a normal distribution, the mean value is appropriate and will provide an average of all data values. If your data has a skewed distribution, the median will be a more appropriate measure than the mean. This is because the median is less affected by extreme values. If your data contains frequently occurring values, the mode will be an appropriate measure to use.

Example: In a sample of five subjects, their body weights were measured as: 70, 70, 70, 70, and 200 kg. The central tendency values are: mean: 96; median: 70; mode: 70. In this case, the median and mode are most representative of the entire data set, whereas the mean value is not.

The choice of central tendency measures the following:

- Data set one: 10, 20, 30, 40, 40; mean value is suitable = 28.
- Data set two: 10, 20, 30, 40, 50, 60; median value is suitable = 35.
- Data set three: 10, 20, 30, 40, 40; mode value is suitable = 40.

Data	Choice of central tendency
Normal distribution (interval/ratio)	Mean
A not normal distribution (interval/ratio)	Median
Ordinal	Median
Nominal	Mode

ASK YOURSELF
▪ What are the four types of measurement scales? ▪ What is a bell-shaped data distribution? ▪ What is *positive skewness*? ▪ What is *kurtosis*? ▪ What are *U-shaped* and *inverted U-shaped data distributions*? ▪ When do you need to perform a normality test? ▪ What does a box plot display? ▪ What is *homogeneity of variance*? What test is used to determine homogeneity of variance? ▪ What is a central tendency? Give examples of when you use mean, median, or mode.

CHAPTER 7

Measurements

TOPIC OUTLINE

- Range
- Standard deviation
- Standard error of the mean
- Coefficient of variation
- Z-score
- T-score
- Confidence interval
- Calculation of CI
- Odds and odds ratio
- Probability
- Relative risk ratio
- Cumulative incidence
- Risk difference
- Hazard ratios

There are endless tools used to measure medical or biomedical data. You may find them in different research articles you read in the literature. These tools should serve the purpose of addressing your research questions and aims.

Range

The *range* is related to the distance between endpoints in a distribution. In other words, the range is the difference between the lowest and highest values in a distribution.

For example, for scores of 3, 4, 5, 6, 7, 8, 9, the Range = Highest Score – Lowest Score, 9 - 3 = 6.

Because the range presents the two most extreme values, it can be a poor indicator of the total data distribution in a data set and does not indicate the data in between. As such, the presentation of the range is often combined with other measurements such as mean and standard deviation.

Example:

The bone mineral density results in 101 patients with Crohn's disease

	Mean ± SD	Range
Spine T-score (young – adult matched)	-0.9 ± 1.3	-4.2 to 1.9
Spine Z-score (age-and weight-matched)	-0.55 ± 1.21	-3.1 to 2.7

The table above has two columns: "Mean ± SD" and "Range." The information in both columns provides the mean value, data distribution, and extreme values, giving an appropriate representation of data variability. On the other hand, a presentation of the range value alone would be inappropriate and leave an unclear picture of the data variability.

Standard Deviation

Standard deviation (SD) represents a within-group individual distribution. SD can also be presented as the Greek letter sigma σ or the Latin letter *s*. SD is a measure used to quantify the variation or dispersion of a set of data values. Therefore, SD indicates the distance an observation falls from the sample mean.

Example:

Group one	Group two
28, 29, 30, 31, 32	10, 20, 30, 40, 50
Mean: 30	Mean: 30
Range: 28 - 32	Range: 10 - 50
SD is small	SD is large

The above table shows two data groups with the same mean value (30). However, the range and standard deviation are smaller in group one than in group two. Therefore, the distribution variance is smaller in group two than in group one. Another way to describe this is that standard deviation indicates how separated the data is. Therefore, the group with a smaller SD will have less dispersed data.

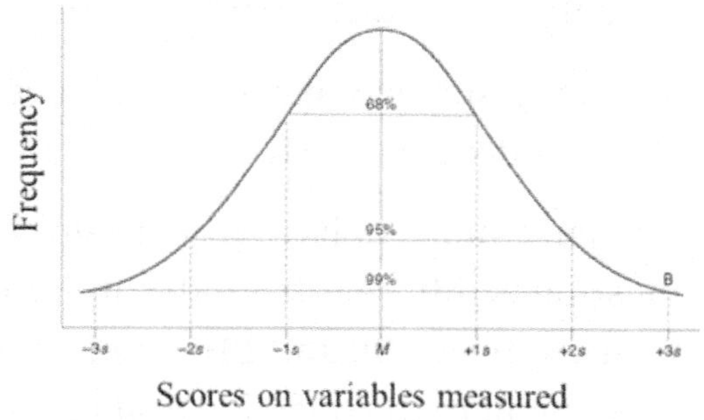

In a normal distribution curve, standard deviation has a particular meaning:

- One standard deviation of the mean covers 68% of the data measured.

- Two standard deviations of the mean covers 95% of the data measured.
- Three standard deviations of the mean covers 99% of the data measured.

Example 1:

M ± SD is 100 ± 10. The data is distributed normally.

The interpretation is that 68% of the data should have scores between 90 and 110, 95% of the data should have scores between 80 and 120, and 99% of the data should have scores between 70 and 130 (within three standard deviations of the mean).

Example 2:

Application of the normal curve and standard deviation.

In two hundred subjects, the average systolic blood pressure is 100 mmHg. The standard deviation is 10 mmHg. A normality test revealed that the data is in a normal distribution.

Question 1: How many subjects have a score between 90 and 110? *Answer:* 68%: 0.68 x 200 = 136.

Question 2: How many subjects have a score greater than 110? *Answer:* This question is different from the above question. The above question asks between 90 and 110, indicating a two-tailed distribution. However, here the question is about a score greater than 110. It is a one-tailed distribution. Therefore the calculation is (0.32 x 200)/2 = 32.

Standard Error of the Mean

The *standard error of the mean* (SEM) measures the variability. It estimates how far the sample means likely are from the population mean. It emphasizes the sample but not individual observations. SEM reflects the variability between sample means.

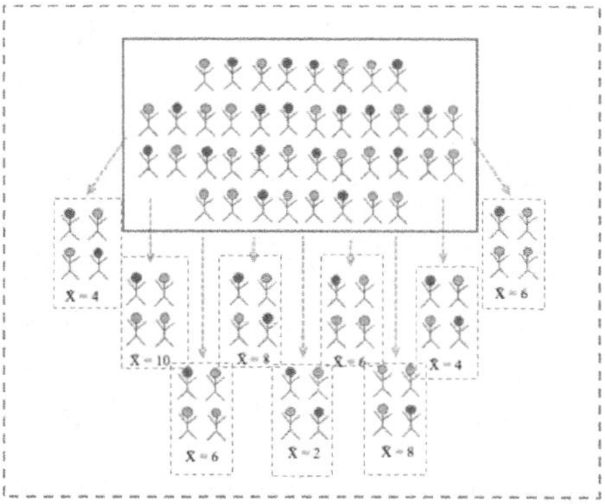

Suppose an overall population comprises different samples. (See figure above.) Then, we can analyze these samples for the mean and standard error of the mean.

SEM is the standard deviation divided by the square root of the sample size.

Interpretation of SEM: SEM measures how representative the sample means are likely to be of the population. When we use samples, they can be seen as inferential statistics. Consequently, sampling distributions in different regions and repeated sampling are necessary to represent the entire population. SEM is an essential part of this process.

Using sample means to estimate population means is inaccurate when the SEM is large. This is because the sample means based on SEM calculation do not reflect individual observations.

Coefficient of Variation

The coefficient of variation (CV) compares the variabilities between two or more data distributions. The larger the CV, the greater the dispersion.

Can you compare CVs when they have different units? Yes, the CV can be used to compare variables with different units, e.g., the variability between sexes (males and females) or between two different diseases.

The formula for the CV is:

CV = (SD/M) x 100

or (standard deviation/mean) * 100

When do you need to use the coefficient of variation?

- To determine the most efficient criteria to be used in a study.
- To aid in selecting the method for a study in an experimental design.
- To allow for meaningful comparisons between two or more magnitudes of variation, even if they have different means or different measurement scales.

Example 1:

Body weight of 100 people: Male mean = 70 kg, SD = 5 kg; female mean = 65 kg, SD =3 kg

Male CV = (5/70) x 100 = 7.1%;

Female CV = (3/65) x 100 = 4.6%.

Interpretation: Male body weight has a greater variation compared to female body weight.

Example 2:

Researchers want to determine which test is more reliable (in terms of minor variation) before launching a large study.

The tests are an extraversion personality (EV) test and another intelligence quotient (IQ) test.

Pilot studies show that EV has a mean value of 50 and a standard deviation of 10. On the other hand, the IQ has a mean value of 100 and a standard deviation of 15.

The calculated CV is 20% for EV and 15% for IQ. Therefore, the answer is that IQ is more reliable.

Example 3:

Coefficient of variation to show variability:

		BMI (kg/m2)	
Year	Mean	SD	CV (%)
1965	21.73	1.98	9.11
1995	21.97	2.76	12.56
2010	22.94	3.63	15.82

This table shows that the CV in BMI has been increasing for about two decades, indicating that this trait's variability in each cohort has increased over time. The data were extracted from a paper (Lipowicz et al., 2015).

Z-Score

A Z-score measures how many standard deviations an element is from the population mean. The Z-score shows how far away a score is from the mean. A Z-score can be placed on a normal distribution curve.

The formulation for calculating a Z-score is Z = [i – M(p)]/SD(p)

Abbreviations: i = individual score; M(p) = population mean; and SD(p) = population standard deviation.

Example:

Mean population body fat (BF) percentage = 25%, SD = 5. Debbie is 18%; Jenny is 35%. What would the Z-scores be for Debbie and Jenny?

Debbie: Z = (18 - 25)/5 = -1.4; Jenny: Z = (35 - 25)/5 = 2.0.

The Z-scores indicate the exact position of the raw score in population distribution. For example, Debbie's Z-score of -1.4 means that Debbie's body fat percentage (BF%) is lower than the population's BF% by 1.4 standard deviations. Jenny's Z-score of two means that Jenny's BF% is greater than the population's BF% by two standard deviations.

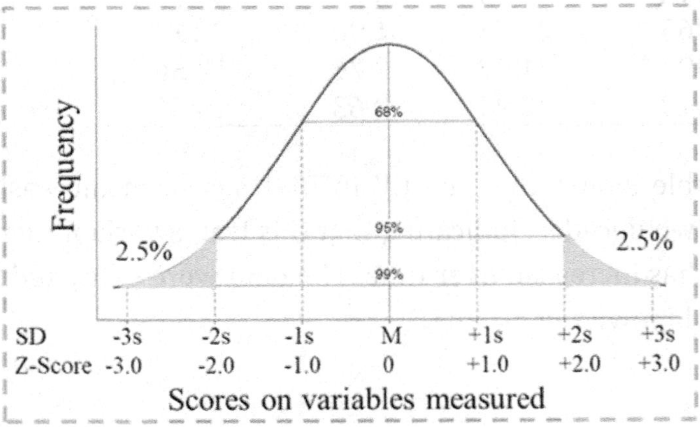

T- Score

The T-score measures how many standard deviations an element is from the sample mean. It is a comparison within subgroup data.

- Calculation of T-score = [i – M(s)]/SD(s)
- Abbreviations: i = individual score; M(s) = the sample mean; SD(s) = the sample standard deviation.

Example:

The mean sample grip strength = 40.0 kg, SD = 3.0. The mean flexibility = 30.0 cm, SD = 4.0.

Jeff: grip = 45 kg; flexibility = 25 cm; What would the T-scores be for Jeff's grip strength and flexibility? Calculation: grip strength: T = (45 – 40)/3 = 1.67. Flexibility: T = (25 – 30)/4 = - 1.25.

Question: Which is the better score for Jeff?

Answer: The T-score indicates the exact position of the raw score in sample distribution. Jeff's grip strength is 1.67 standard deviations above the sample mean. In contrast, his flexibility is 1.25 standard deviations below the sample mean. Therefore, Jeff is strong in grip strength but not very flexible compared to the sample.

Application of T-Score

The T-score is your bone density differing from the bone density of an average healthy young adult of your sex. *Young adult* refers to someone thirty years of age. A T-score helps diagnose bone density. The World Health Organization's criteria for diagnosing osteoporosis use bone-mineral-density measurements. The below table shows the following:

The T-score is used to compare you with a sample size ≤ 30. A T-score is a standard deviation. Your T-score is your bone mineral density (BMD) as a standard deviation from the mean. A dual-energy X-ray absorptiometry (DXA) machine can scan your bone density and report T-scores, showing how much higher or lower your bone density is than that of a healthy thirty-year-old.

The WHO criteria

T-Score	Diagnosis
≥ - 1.0	Normal
< -1.0 and > -2.5	Osteopenia
≤ -2.5	Osteoporosis
≤ -2.5 or lower+fractures	Severe osteoporosis

- T-Score is ≥ -1.0, indicating a healthy bone density.
- T-Score is < -1.0 and > -2.5, indicating osteopenia.
- T-Score is ≤ -2.5, indicating osteoporosis.

You can also compare your bone density with the average bone density of people your age and gender in the population, which is a Z-score.

Example 1:

An exercise physiologist wants to compare John's tibial bone density with the national average tibial bone density. What test should they choose? What values should they report? Z-score test; outcome comparing Z-scores.

Example 2:

An exercise physiologist wants to compare John's tibial bone density with his male classmates' average tibial bone density. What test should they choose? What values should they report? T-score test; outcome comparing T-scores.

Summary of Calculations of Z-score and T-Score

Z- Score	T-Score
Know population standard deviation, SD(p) Know population mean, M(p) Generally n > 30 Q: individual (i) vs. population Z= [i – M(p)]/SD(p)	Do not know population standard deviation, SD(s) Know sample mean, M(s), sample SD, SD(S) Generally n < 30 Q: individual (i) vs. sample or subgroup T= [i –M(s)]/SD(s)

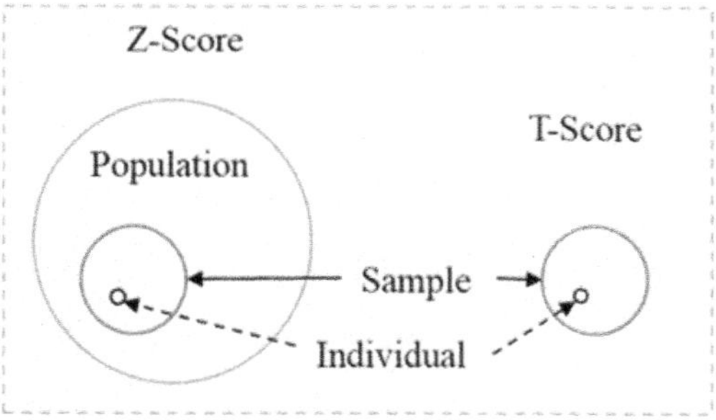

Confidence Interval

A confidence interval (CI) is a range of values in which we are confident our actual value lies.

For example, a 95% CI means that our actual value is in this range. CI is commonly used in the risk and prevalence (OR and RR) reports.

Example:

The mean systolic blood pressure in a group of one hundred people is 120 mmHg (95% confidence interval, CI: 90, 140). Therefore, the interpretation is that ninety-five subjects will have a blood pressure measurement between 90 and 140 mmHg.

Confident in Determining the CI

The higher the % of confidence, the wider the CI range. e.g., n = 100. When you increase confidence, the CI range increases.

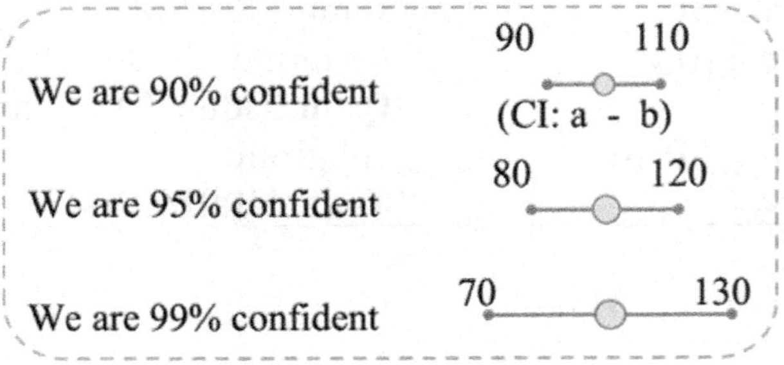

Example:

A 90% confidence range is 90–110. If the confidence level increases to 95%, the range increases to 80–120. Therefore, the more confident (99% > 95% > 90%), the larger confidence interval will be.

Confidence Interval and Critical Value

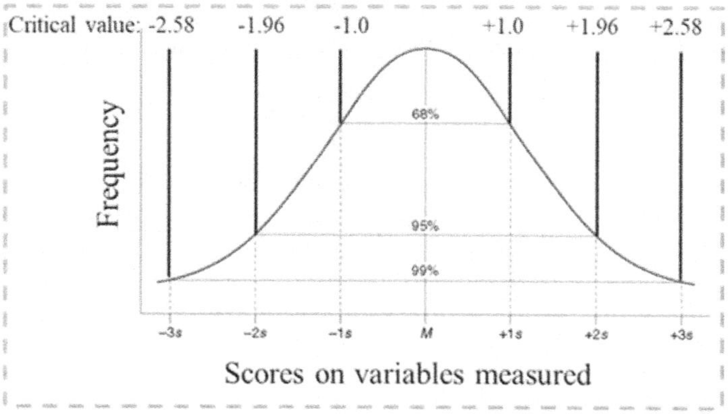

The figure shows that as the CI increases in a normal distribution, so does the CI range. This is reflected in the critical value i.e., 68%: -1.0 to +1.0; 95%: -1.96 to +1.96.

The difference between a critical value and an alpha value: An *alpha value* is a significance level. If the alpha value is 0.05, 95% of the data is covered. A CI is a range of values we are sure of out of our actual values. A confidence interval of 95% [95% CI] has a critical value of ± 1.96. A confidence interval of 68% [68% CI] has a critical value of ± 1.0.

The difference between standard deviation and confidence interval: A *standard deviation* represents data distribution, for example, 40 ± 10 with a data range of 30 to 50. The CI value relies on the critical value.

Example:

Here is a calculation of a mean value of 40 with a 95% or 99% confidence interval.

Calculation of CI

Provides an expected upper and lower limit value

What is the 95% CI?	What is the 99% CI?
CI = mean(M) ± (SE x confidence level$_{\text{(Critical value)}}$)	
M = 40, SE =1.46,	
Critical value = ± 1.96	**Critical value** = ± 2.58
CI=40 ± (1.46 x 1.96) = 40 ± 2.86 = *37.14 to 42.86*	= 40 ± (1.46 x 2.58) = 40 ± 3.77 = *36.23 to 43.77*
95% confident that this interval contains the target population mean	99% confident that this interval contains the target population mean

For a 95% confidence interval, it is 40 ± 2.86 = 37.14–42.86. The report is 40 [37.14, 42.86, 95% CI]. We are sure that our value is between 37.14 and 42.86 with 95% confidence.

Odds and Odds Ratio

Odds are the number of events that produce the outcome of interest to the number of events that do not.

Example: The odds of rolling a two on a six-sided dice is one to five (1:5). This is because there is a single event (rolling a two); however, five events do not result in the outcome of interest (rolling a 1, 3, 4, 5, or 6).

Odds are a measure of *association* between an exposure and an outcome (cases and controls)

Odds: 1/5

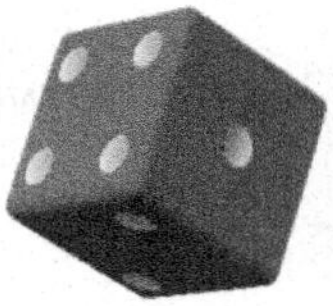

What about coming up as 2? 1/5

Incidence

What about coming up as 4 or 5? 2/4

Odds ratio

- An odds ratio (OR) represents the odds that an outcome will occur given a particular exposure compared to the odds of the outcome occurring in the absence of that exposure (i.e., cases and controls).
- An OR is a measure of association between a disease and exposure (often using cases and controls).
- Formulation: OR = Exposure (diseased/not diseased)/no exposure (diseased/not diseased).

Significance of an OR

- If cases have higher odds of exposure than controls, exposure may increase disease risk.
- If cases have lower odds of exposure than controls, exposure may reduce the risk of disease (i.e., protective effect).
- If cases and controls have equal odds of exposure, exposure is likely not related to disease development.

Interpretation of an OR

- OR = 1, no change in the frequency of exposure among cases.
- OR > 1, increased frequency of exposure among cases.
- OR < 1, decreased frequency of exposure among cases.

When Do You Use OR?

The odds ratio is usually used for risk factors, for example, in a case-control study.

OR Calculation in a Case-Control Study

The odds ratio is a ratio of two odds.

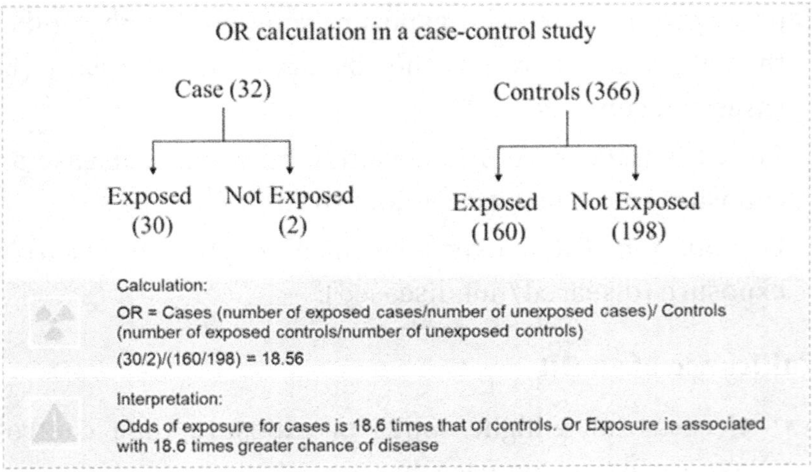

OR Represents the Risk Level

Example: Researchers want to investigate whether or not smoking is a risk factor for the development of lung cancer.

Risk	Disease status	
	Present	Absent
Smoker	*a* 30	*b* 160
Non-smoker	*c* 2	*d* 198

The table shows the data collected, binary data. It shows that 30 smokers developed cancer, 160 smokers did not develop cancer, 200 non-smokers developed cancer, and 198 have no cancer. OR = (30/160)/(2/198) = 18.56

The results show that the chance of lung cancer development is 18.56 times greater for smokers than non-smokers.

SPSS Computer Software Calculates the OR by Logistic Regression

Risk Estimate

	Value	95% Confidence Interval	
		Lower	Upper
Odds Ratio for Exposure cat (smoker / no smoker)	18.563	4.370	78.853
For cohort Disease = cancer	1.176	1.104	1.252
For cohort Disease = no cancer	.063	.015	.261
N of Valid Cases	390		

The risk estimate shows that the odds ratio for exposure to non-exposure is 18.56 (95% CI).

The OR Represents the Sample but Not the Population

The flowchart shows that researchers found twenty-two disease cases and five hundred non-diseased controls in a sample.

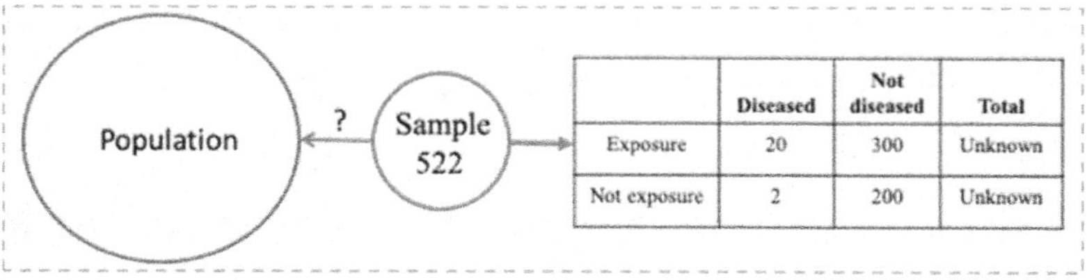

	Diseased	Not diseased	Total
Exposure	20	300	Unknown
Not exposure	2	200	Unknown

The analysis shows that OR = (20/300)/(2/200) = 6.7.

Therefore, the exposure gives a 6.7 times higher risk of developing the disease.

However, we do not know the population size.

Adjusted OR. In many cases, you need to adjust for covariances to provide an adjusted OR value. An example can be found in a previous paper, which adjusted for age, sex, BMI, and fasting glucose (Wang et al., 2013).

Example 1: Odds ratio shows correlations between variables

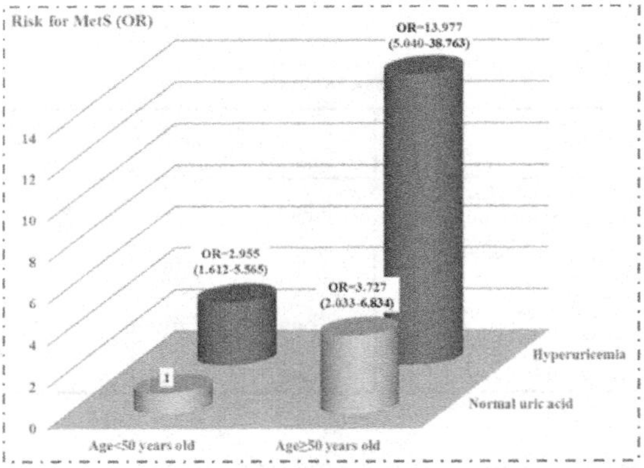

The figure shows the interaction between age, ≥ 50 years or < 50 years, and hyperuricemia for metabolic syndrome. The statistical analysis was a nonparametric test. The odds ratios used a 95% confidence interval. It shows that bipolar patients with hyperuricemia over fifty years old were more prone to developing metabolic syndrome (OR = 14.0, CI95[5.040 - 38.763]). The figure was adapted and modified from our paper (Chen et al., 2018).

Example 2: OR represents the association between the risk factor and outcome

Table:

Associations between WC and HTG with the risk of having hyperuricemia

Variable	OR	95% CI	p
Increased WC	2.128	1.233-4.034	0.007
HTG	1.870	1.112-3.121	0.017

WC: waist circumference, > 90 cm in men, > 80 cm in women; HTG: hypertriglyceridemia, triglycerides > 1.70 mmol/L (150 mg/dL) for men and women. Therefore, there were four groups. They were patients with and without increased WC and healthy controls with and without increased WC.

Report: The hyperuricemia were higher with increased WC (OR = 2.1, CI95[1.2–4.0]) and HTG (OR = 1.9, CI95[1.1–3.1]). The table was adopted with modifications from our paper (Chen et al., 2018).

Probability (*p*)

Statistical decisions are not exact but are made with a probability or chance of being right or wrong.

A probability statement is commonly denoted by the letter *p* and expressed in proportions of 1. A probability of 1 means there is a 100% certainty of an event occurring. A probability of 0 means there is no chance of an event occurring. Therefore, probability statements range from 0 to 1.

Example:

The *p* value is the number of events is divided by the number of possible events.

When flipping a coin once, what is the probability it will come up with tails? $p = 1/2 = 0.5$ or 50%.

When rolling a six-sided dice once, what is the probability of rolling a 3? $p = 1/6 = 0.167$ or 16.7%.

When rolling a six-sided dice once, what is the probability of rolling a 2 or a 5? $p = 2/6 = 0.333$ or 33.3%.

In a standard deck of cards, there are fifty-two cards, with four jacks in a deck. When selecting a card randomly, what is the probability of drawing a jack? $p = 4/52 = 0.077$ or 7.7%.

After performing a statistical test, a probability statement is generated, such as $p < 0.05$ (or the actual p-value). Example: $t = 2.47$, $p < 0.05$, there is significant difference.

What Does $p < 0.05$ Mean?

It means there is less than a 5% chance that the hypothesis is correct for the H_0 (null hypothesis). Or there is a 95% confidence that an H_A (alternative hypothesis) is correct. Therefore, we reject the H_0 (null) hypothesis and accept the H_A (alternative) hypothesis.

Probability Versus Odds

Odds are about incidence, whereas probability is about the prevalence or relative risk.

Example:

Rolling a six-sided dice once, the odds of rolling a 3 is 1 to 5, but the probability is 1 in 6.

When flipping a coin, the odds of landing on tails is 1 to 1, but the probability is 1 in 2.

In a raffle of 10,000 tickets, the odds of a person who has purchased one ticket winning is 1 to 9,999, and the probability is 1 in 10,000.

Therefore, the probability is about the same as the odds when the incidence is rare.

p = The number of ways an event in question can occur divided by the number of possible events.

Probability: 1/6

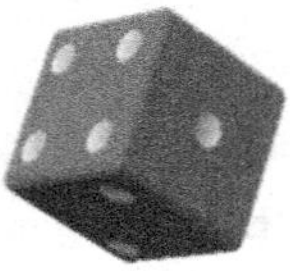

A coin: Heads or tails:

- Prob ½ ; Odds 1/1

Raffle with 10,000 people:

- Prob 1/10,000; Odds 1/9,999

In rare incidence, Prob ~ Odds

Relative Risk Ratio

Relative risk (R) is a ratio of the probabilities of an event in an exposed group.

Relative risk ratio (RR): It is the ratio of the probability of an event in an exposed group to the probability of an event in a non-exposed group.

In this way, RR represents an event risk (e.g., disease) of an exposed group compared to the event risk of a non-exposed group. The RR is a ratio of two probabilities.

		Diseased	Not diseased	Total	Cumulative incidence	RR
Predictor	Exposed	100	1900	2000	100/(100+1900)=5 %	5/0.1 = 50%
	Non-exposed	10	1990	2000	10/(10+1990) =0.1%	

$$RR = \frac{(A/(A+B))}{(C/(C+D))}$$

The figure illustrates an RR as a predictor that a researcher might consider.

Example:

The below table shows how RR is calculated. Here the RR of developing the disease (e.g., lung cancer) is calculated given exposure to smoking. The RR informs us that smokers are 15.8 times more likely to develop the disease of interest than non-smokers.

Risk	Disease status	
	Present	Absent
Smoker	a	b
Non-smoker	c	d

Risk	Disease status	
	Present	Absent
Smoker	30	160
Non-smoker	2	198

RR=[a/(a+b)]/[c/(c+d)] = 15.8

Or in %: Formulation = (RR-1) x 100 = (15.8 -1) x 100 = 148%. The risk of disease is increased by 148%.

The Values of RR

- RR = 1 = No increased risk of an outcome.
- RR = > 1 = Increased risk of an outcome.
- RR = < 1 = Reduced risk of an outcome.
- RR represents x times more or x%.

How large should the RR be for us to be impressed?

- Suggestion: This will depend on the level of evidence acquired.
- In a randomized controlled trial, researchers would be satisfied with a small increase or decrease in risk.
- In a cohort study: RR > 3 should be considered.
- In a case-control study: RR > 4 should be considered.

Baseline Risk

A patient's baseline risk can contribute to the overall risk. Usually, a paper summarizes this risk in a group or population. When an individual RR is considered, the conclusion requires a consideration of the baseline risk.

The importance of RR also depends on the baseline risk.

Example:

When a paper reports RR = 3.0, the likelihood of developing the outcome is three times more likely if exposed to *X*.

If the baseline risk is 30%, a RR of 3.0 means the total risk increases to 90%, given exposure to *X*. So, in this case, the RR is likely important.

However, if the baseline risk is 0.1%, then a RR of 3.0 means the total risk increases to 0.3%. So, in this case, the RR may not be that important.

Considering Individual Baseline Risk

Example:

Researchers investigated the effect of combined estrogen and progestin therapy on the risk of cardiovascular disease (Grodstein et al., 1996).

Based on a previous study, from 431 cases who have never used estrogen or progestin, RR = 1, the baseline, table 2 (Grodstein et al., 1996). From the eight cases using estrogen and progestin, RR = 0.39. Therefore, the risk of CVD is reduced by 61% [(1 - 0.39) x 100] in cases using estrogen and progestin.

Lisa saw this paper. She was diagnosed with metabolic syndrome, having an estimated 20% baseline risk of developing coronary artery disease (CAD). If Lisa was on hormone therapy using estrogen and progestin (E/P), what would be her estimated probability of CAD later in life?

CVD risk: 0.2 x 0.39 = 0.078; 7.8%; reduced by 20% - 7.8% = 12.2%

Comparing an Odds Ratio and Relative Risk Ratio in a Rare Disease

An *odds ratio* (OR) is the relative exposure distribution commonly used concerning a risk factor. If the disease is rare (<10%), the OR is almost the same as the relative risk ratio (RR).

The below table 1 shows the OR = (20/300)/(2/200) = 6.67. The risk of disease is 6.67 times higher when exposed to the risk factor. RR = (20/320)/(2/202) = 6.313. The relative risk is 6.313 times higher than the unexposed group.

The OR is not much different from RR.

Table 1	Disease	No disease
Exposure	20	300
Non-exposure	2	200

Table 2	Disease	No disease
Exposure	60	300
Non-exposure	2	200

Comparing an odds ratio and relative risk ratio in a common disease

If the disease is common (> 10%), the OR exaggerates the strength of an estimated association.

The above table 2 shows the OR = (60/300)/(2/200) = 20. Risk ratio = (60/360)/(2/202) = 16.83.

The OR is very different from the RR.

Example:

The table shows the prevalence (%) and relative risk (odds ratio) of smoking among students in four schools.

School	No	Smokers (%)	Odds ratio (OR)	Adjusted OR
1	639	19.3	1*	1*
2	392	15.8	0.78 (0.56-1.10)#	0.61 (0.40-0.94)#
3	353	34.4	2.2 (1.63-2.96)	1.48 (1.01-2.18)
4	461	25.2	1.41 (1.05-1.89)	1.06 (0.73-1.53)

*: Reference school. #: 95% confidence intervals obtained by logistic regression. The data were adopted with modifications from a paper (Azevedo et al., 1999).

Cumulative Incidence

Cumulative incidence (CuI) is calculated by dividing the new cases (e.g., of disease) by the total number of individuals in the population at risk for a specific period. Using CuI, the proportion of a population at risk of disease may be predicted during a specific period.

Cumulative incidence can be calculated in a cohort or randomized controlled trial. However, we see that a cohort study frequently calculates cumulative incidence.

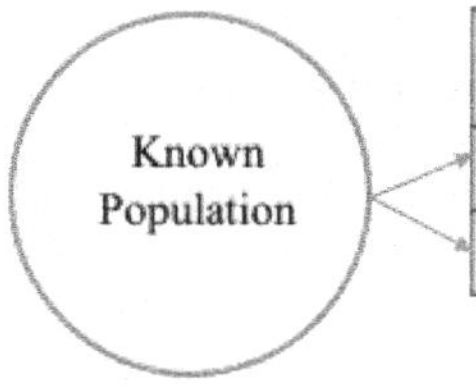

	Diseased	Not diseased	Total	Cumulative incidence
Exposed	100	1900	2000	100/(100+1900)=5%
Non-exposed	10	1990	2000	10/(10+1990) =0.1%

In a cohort study, we can calculate cumulative incidence. This is because the overall population is known, which is considered in the study design. The total number of diseased and non-diseased cases is known for both the exposed and non-exposed groups. The table above shows a 5% cumulative incidence in the exposed group. In the non-exposed group, there is a 0.1% cumulative incidence.

Why Can't We Calculate Cumulative Incidence in a Case-Control Study?

An odds ratio is used in a case-control study; however, we cannot calculate cumulative incidence because we do not know the total number of new cases in a given period.

The total number of exposed and non-exposed subjects is unknown since sampling was done using a case-control design (retrospectively). The information from non-diseased controls allows us to estimate the exposure distribution in the source population; however, we don't know the denominators (totals).

Risk difference

Risk difference (RD) is the difference in the risk of an outcome (e.g., disease) between exposed and non-exposed groups. Risk difference is also called *attributable risk* or *excess risk*. RD is calculated by subtracting the cumulative incidence (CuI) in the non-exposed group from the cumulative incidence in the exposed group. RD measures the effectiveness of risk reduction or promotion, comparing absolute differences between the two groups.

Risk Difference (RD) = $CuI_e - Cui_u$

Where CuI_e = the cumulative incidence among the exposed subjects.

Where CuI_u = the cumulative incidence among non-exposed subjects.

RD focuses on the absolute effect of the risk factor or the excess risk of disease in those who have the risk factor compared with those who don't.

	Diseased	Not diseased	Total	Cumulative incidence	RD
Exposed	100	1,900	2,000	100/(100+1,900)=5%	5-0.1=4.9
Non-exposed	10	1,990	2,000	10/(10+1,990)=0.1%	

Interpretation of Risk Difference

The report can describe the excess risk in the group exposed to the risk factor by converting percentages to fractions.

Example:

The infection rates in diabetes patients versus non-diabetes patients:

CuI with diabetes = 6.3% = 63/1000.

CuI without diabetes = 1.3% = 13/1000.

Risk difference = 50/1000 = 5/100.

An interpretation is that diabetes subjects have five extra infection cases per one hundred subjects than those who do not have diabetes.

Relative Risk Versus Risk Difference

Relative risk gives a percentage value, while *risk difference* gives an attribute value.

Example:

Researchers want to find how effective fecal blood testing is as a screening test to identify colorectal cancer.

- *Relative risk (RR):* The study found that people over the age of forty who were screened had a 31% reduction in death (i.e., RR = 0.69; 69%) from colorectal cancer compared to people who were not screened. In other words, those who were screened had 0.69 times (reduction) in the risk of death from colorectal cancer.
- *Risk difference (RD):* The incidence of death in the screened group was five per one thousand people, and the incidence of death in the unscreened group was eight per one thousand. In other words, screening may have saved three lives per one thousand people screened (8 reduced to 5 is a 38% reduction).

A 38% reduction sounds like a lot, but when you consider that the risk difference is three per one thousand people, it is easier to understand the impact.

Rate Difference Versus Risk Difference

Rate difference: A measure of the strength of the association between a risk factor and an outcome (e.g., disease), e.g., odds ratio, risk ratio, rate ratio.

Risk difference: A risk difference (RD) is an absolute risk. RD is usually used when investigating the population health impact of a risk factor. It focuses on the number of patients that could potentially be prevented by eliminating the risk factor.

Hazard Ratio

Hazard ratio (HR) is a survival analysis that can be used in cohort studies and randomized controlled trials. HR is often reported in a time-to-event analysis.

HR = Hazard in treatment /Hazard in control

The relative risk (R) does not account for the time-to-event but the event's occurrence at the end of the study. HR is frequently interpreted as relative risk (or risk ratio), but they are not technically equivalent because HR accounts for the time.

- HR = 1, event rates are the same as controls.
- HR = 2, twice as many subjects in the treated group having an event compared to the controls at any given time.
- HR = 0.5, half as many subjects in the treated group having an event compared to the controls at any given time.

Cumulative Incidence, Risk Difference, and Risk Ratio

For example, we assume when evaluating the risk of stomach pain after taking metformin, the cumulative incidence is:

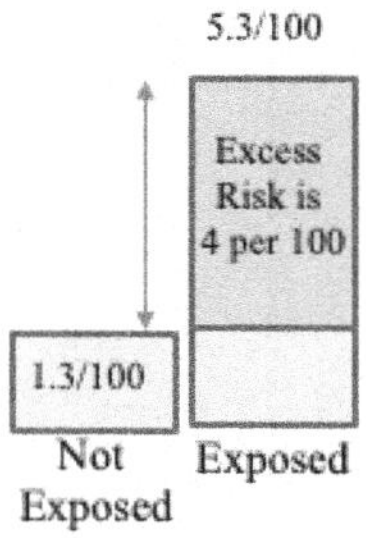

- 5.3% in the exposed group (taking metformin).
- 1.3% in the not exposed group (not taking metformin).
- Therefore, the baseline CuI is 1.3%.

- The risk difference is 5.3 - 1.3 = 4 per 100.
- The risk ratio is (5.3/100)/(1.3/100) = 4.1.

ASK YOURSELF
▪ What are the similarities and the differences between standard deviation and standard error of the mean? ▪ When should you use the measurement of coefficient of variation? ▪ What are the similarities and the differences between Z-score and T-score? ▪ What is the confidence interval? ▪ What does the critical value 1.96 mean in the confidence interval range? ▪ How is the confidence interval calculated? ▪ When is a cumulative incidence measure required? ▪ Why can cumulative incidence not be calculated in a case-control study? ▪ What does the odds ratio measure? What is the significance of the odds ratio? ▪ What does relative risk represent? How is relative risk calculated? ▪ What are the differences between odds and probability? ▪ Why is it necessary to assess the baseline risk of your patients before a conclusion can be drawn from the RR value?

CHAPTER 8

Hypothesis, *P*-Value, and Errors

TOPIC OUTLINE

- Research hypothesis
- Statistical hypothesis
- *P*-value
- Adjusted *p*-value
- Type I and type II errors

A hypothesis aims to introduce a research question or propose an expected result. The research hypothesis is a statement created by the researcher. It should be a specific and testable prediction. Constructing an idea or hypothesis based on background research with further exploration is always helpful.

All quantitative studies should begin with a formulated hypothesis. A hypothesis should be quantifiable and specific and predict a particular size relationship or effect.

A hypothesis is used to speculate on the outcome of a research or experiment.

Examples:

Swimmers have better flexibility than runners.

Estrogen users have superior muscle composition due to the hormonal and metabolic effects of estrogen and, as a result, have more muscle strength and increased physical function.

Hypothesis Criteria

It relates to the research topic.

It has both an independent variable that can be manipulated and a dependent variable.

It is testable by a method.

It has an expected outcome.

Hypothesis Types

Simple Hypothesis versus Complex Hypothesis:

In a *simple hypothesis*, one independent variable predicts one dependent variable. A *complex hypothesis* may predict the relationship between two or more independent variables.

Directional Hypothesis versus Non-Directional Hypothesis:

A *directional hypothesis* has an expected direction based on the previous studies determining the relationship between variables. When the outcome contradicts the previous research, a *non-directional hypothesis* can be applied.

Association Hypothesis versus Causal Hypothesis:

An *association hypothesis* has an interdependent relationship between variables. A *causal hypothesis* predicts an effect on the dependent variable due to the manipulation of the independent variable.

Statistical Hypothesis:

A *statistical hypothesis* concerns the parameters of a probability supporting the hypothesis.

The statistical hypothesis contains the null hypothesis and the alternative hypothesis. A *null hypothesis* (H_0) proposes no statistical significance in a set of given observations. An *alternative hypothesis* is that the researcher anticipates a difference between variables.

Null hypothesis (H_0)	Alternative hypothesis (H_A)
It is hypothesized that: There is no difference or relationship We compare two population means (M) H_0: M1 - M2 = 0; M1= M2 There is no difference between the two population means. It is assumed to be true until proven otherwise.	The null hypothesis (H0) stated that there is no difference; however, if this is not true, what has to be true? H_A: M1-M2 $\neq$ 0; M1$\neq$M2 There is a difference between the two population means.

H_0 and H_A hypothesis and alpha value L:

- H_0: M1:M2:M3, $p > 0.05$, accept H_0, and reject H_A.
- H_0: M1:M2:M3, $p < 0.05$, reject H_0, and accept H_A.

Example:

Here is a statistical hypothesis. A researcher hypothesizes no difference in the fasting blood glucose levels between the university "n" students and their city population, which is 6.8 mmol/L.

Testable Hypothesis

Example 1: Patients with type 2 diabetes have a higher incidence of cardiovascular disease than healthy subjects. Test a group of people with type 2 diabetes against a diabetes-free group and determine the percentage of cardiovascular disease within each group. The test can be done and repeated.

Example 2: Smokers are more likely to develop lung infections than non-smokers. Test a group of smokers against non-smokers and determine the percentage of lung infections within each group.

Non-Testable Hypothesis

Example 1: "It is irrelevant if subjects have type 2 diabetes." This hypothesis is not testable. What is "irrelevant"? What is the outcome? The hypothesis is vague and cannot be tested.

Example 2: "Smoking could cause hypertension." This hypothesis is not testable because the word "could" is unclear and difficult to prove.

Example 3: "Hypertension has better outcomes than depression." This hypothesis is vague and not testable because the two conditions are incompatible and cannot be compared. We are not clear on what we are trying to prove.

Example 4: A hypothesis needs to be specific and testable: Is it possible to design a quantitative research project based on the hypothesis that breastfed babies have a lower incidence of illness than babies given formula? This is not a workable hypothesis because it does not specify what disease, how to feed, how long, or what the risk is. A better quantitative hypothesis will be that babies who are exclusively breastfed for three months or more have a lower incidence of hospital admissions for gastroenteritis by at least 30 percent over the first year of life.

p-value

The *p*-value, or *probability value,* refers to the likelihood that your data occurred by random chance (i.e., the null hypothesis is true). A *p*-value validates the hypothesis against outcome data. Usually, we use $p > 0.05$, the probability that the null hypothesis is true.

How to Accept or Reject the H_0 Hypothesis

We accept the H_0 as being true when we are 95% certain that a result is genuine. This refers to a 95% confidence, with an α value of 0.05.

If $p > 0.05$, there is no statistically significant difference between the two population means. Therefore, we accept the H_0.

If $p < 0.05$, there is a statistically significant difference between the two population means. Therefore, we reject the H_0.

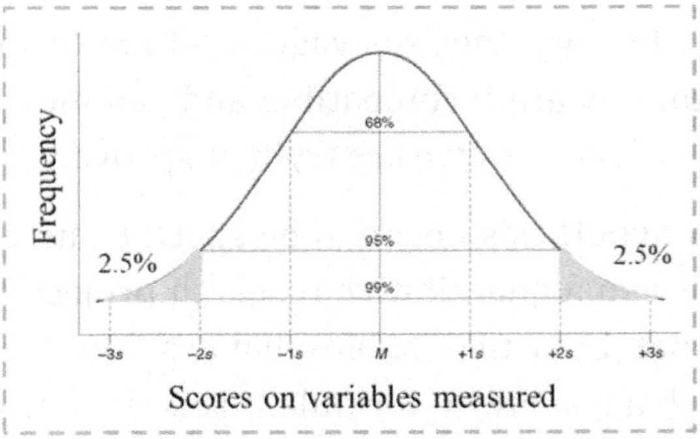

The figure above shows data in a normal distribution with an alpha value set at 0.05 with 2.5% on each side (two-tailed).

What Does a *P*-Value in Two-Tailed or One-Tailed Tests Mean?

The two-tailed test examines the effect in two directions, i.e., positive and negative. The one-tailed test examines the effect in one direction, either positive or negative.

Example:

The *p*-value in a two-tailed test	The *p*-value in a one-tailed test
Hypothesis: Does this exercise protocol affect body weight? A two-tailed T-test should be used. 0.25% + 95% + 0.25%	Hypothesis: Does this exercise protocol lower body weight? A one-tailed T-test should be used. 5% + 95%

General rule: A two-tailed T-test should be used unless there is a strong case for the one-tailed version.

Do You Choose a Two-Tailed or a One-Tailed Test with the Following Example?

Example:

An exercise physiologist wants to design an exercise protocol to affect body weight. However, they do not specify if the protocol will increase or reduce body weight; therefore, a two-tailed test will need to be used.

Alternatively, they want to test whether the application of this exercise protocol reduces body weight. The body weight reduction is specified in the question; therefore, a one-tailed T-test should be used.

The choice between a two- and one-tailed test will depend on the study's hypothesis.

In a research design, we should define the *p*-value, power of the test, confidence interval, and effect size if possible.

Adjusted *P*-Value

The *adjusted* p-*value* is used in multiple comparisons in ANOVA. This analysis aims to determine which factors within multiple comparisons are significantly different. An adjusted *p*-value applies when the same *p*-value is used for multiple comparisons on the same cases and controls.

Example: A comparison between case and control groups uses an independent T-test or chi-square test in genotype and allele frequencies. The null hypothesis is rejected if the adjusted *p*-value is less than alpha. This correction aims to prevent a possible type I error.

Bonferroni adjustment or correction: You can divide the original alpha value by the number of comparisons. Then use that value as an adjusted *p*-value to determine significance. For example, with alpha set at 0.05 and twenty comparisons, the LSD *p*-value required for significance would be 0.05/20 = 0.0025.

TABLE 2. CLINICAL CHARACTERISTICS OF MEDICARE AND VETERANS HEALTH ADMINISTRATION (VHA) PATIENTS ADMITTED FOR ACUTE MYOCARDIAL INFARCTION.*

VARIABLE	MEDICARE PATIENTS (N=29,249)	VHA PATIENTS (N=2486)	P VALUE†
Coexisting condition — no. (%)			
Congestive heart failure	5,939 (20.3)	507 (20.4)	0.92
Prior myocardial infarction	9,695 (33.1)	899 (36.2)	0.002
Percutaneous transluminal coronary angioplasty	2,264 (7.7)	152 (6.1)	0.003
Coronary-artery bypass graft surgery	4,968 (17.0)	447 (18.0)	0.21
Hypertension	16,759 (57.3)	1598 (64.3)	<0.001
Diabetes	8,489 (29.0)	866 (34.8)	<0.001
Diabetes treated with insulin	1,920 (6.6)	271 (10.9)	<0.001
Asthma or chronic obstructive pulmonary disease	6,864 (23.5)	768 (30.9)	<0.001
Stroke	4,154 (14.2)	508 (20.4)	<0.001
Cirrhosis or hepatic failure	153 (0.5)	17 (0.7)	0.29
HIV infection or AIDS	17 (0.1)	3 (0.1)	0.23
Cancer	960 (3.3)	63 (2.5)	0.04
Immunosuppression	583 (2.0)	106 (4.3)	<0.001
Peptic ulcer	4,217 (14.4)	416 (16.7)	0.002
Dementia	1,413 (4.8)	178 (7.2)	<0.001
Terminal illness	139 (0.5)	12 (0.5)	0.96
Order for limitation of resuscitation	4,442 (15.2)	465 (18.7)	<0.001
Body-mass index measured — no. (%)	25,607 (87.5)	1905 (76.6)	<0.001
Body-mass index	26.1±4.5	26.7±5.1	<0.001

*Plus–minus values are means ±SE. HIV denotes human immunodeficiency virus, and AIDS the acquired immunodeficiency syndrome. The body-mass index is the weight in kilograms divided by the square of the height in meters.

†P values less than 0.001 were deemed significant, after the Bonferroni adjustment.

The table above shows how to adjust the *p*-value in a post hoc analysis (Petersen et al., 2000). Given multiple testings, $p < 0.05$ may not be suitable to determine statistical significance. Therefore, researchers used the Bonferroni adjustment on each test to reduce a potential type I error. Here, $p < 0.001$ is used for statistical significance. (0.05/19 items = 0.0026; therefore, choosing 0.001 is conservative).

Type I Error

A type I error means that the H_0 is rejected when it is true: Null is true: type I error false positive. A false positive occurs when a researcher incorrectly rejects a true null hypothesis. The probability of making a type I error is the alpha level.

A researcher may alter the alpha value from 0.05 to 0.01, preventing a type I error. This is because an alpha value of 0.01 is more stringent than an alpha value of 0.05.

Type II Error

A type II error means that the H_0 is accepted when it is false: Null is false: correct effect exists. It is a false negative conclusion. The researcher falsely concludes that the statistical difference was due to sampling error when it was a real effect.

The probability of making a type II error is related to the beta (β) level (directly related to power). Statisticians refer to this concept as the *power of a hypothesis test*. The quantity (1 – β) is the statistical power. Usually, researchers use a study power of 0.8 or 80%, which would make β 0.2 or the chance of creating a type II error 20%. Thus, when power increases, β or the possibility of having a type II error will decrease.

Example: A rapid antigen test (RAT) shows that you were positive for COVID-19. In fact, you did not have a COVID-19 infection. This is a type I error. Conversely, you are infected by the virus, but the RAT is negative. This is a type II error.

		Reality	
		Not reject H_0	Reject H_0
Study finding	Positive H_0 is true	True positive	False positive ***Type I error*** α
	Negative H_0 is false	False negative ***Type II error*** β	True negative

Significance Levels and the Alpha Value

- An α level of 0.05 ($p = 0.05$) means that there is a five in one hundred chance of rejecting the H_0 when it is true.
- An α level of 0.01 means there is a one in one hundred chance of rejecting the H_0 when it is true.

ASK YOURSELF
▪ What are the four major types of hypotheses? ▪ What are the criteria to be considered when proposing a hypothesis? ▪ How do you know whether to accept or reject the H_0 hypothesis? ▪ When do you use a one-tailed T-test? ▪ When do you use an adjusted *p*-value? ▪ What is the difference between type I and type II errors? ▪ How are type I and type II errors controlled in research?

CHAPTER 9

Parametric Test

TOPIC OUTLINE

- T-test
- Pearson correlation coefficient
- Coefficient of determination
- Coefficient of non-determination
- Correlation matrix
- Simple linear regression
- Multiple linear regression
- Logistic regression
- Analysis of variance (ANOVA)
- One-way ANOVA
- Post hoc analysis
- One-way repeated measures ANOVA
- Two-way ANOVA
- Two-way repeated-measures ANOVA
- Analysis of covariance

Parametric tests analyze the interval and ratio data with the underlying assumptions that the data is about the population distribution from which researchers obtain samples, the data have a normal distribution, and the data have homogeneity of variances and linear relationships.

Parametric tests include the T-test, analysis of variance (ANOVA), and Pearson coefficient of correlation.

T-Test

A T-test aims to determine if there is a significant difference between the means of the two groups. The two groups should vary in independent variables, and the outcome or dependent variable should be measured.

Assumptions of a T-test are as follows:

- Sample or population data have a normal distribution.
- There is similar variance.
- Data is continuous.

The Differences Between Standard Deviation and Standard Error of the Mean

Standard Deviation

- It shows how much individuals within the same sample differ from the sample mean.
- It does not describe the accuracy of the sample mean.
- It describes the variability of individual values.
- Mean ± SD.

Standard Error of the Mean

- It shows how close the sample mean is to the population mean.
- It describes the accuracy of the sample mean.
- It does not describe the variability of individual values.
- Mean ± SE.

Testing the Differences Between Two Groups

You can use the T-test, Z-score, and T-score to analyze the differences between the two groups.

T-Test:

This includes one sample T-tests, independent T-tests, and paired T-tests.

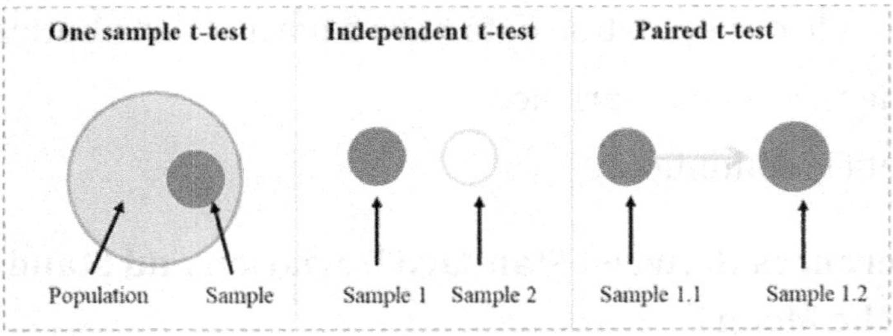

One Sample T-Test

The one-sample T-test analyses the difference between the means of a sample and the population. The sample is part of the population. (See figure above.)

Example: We assume that the population value of fasting glucose is 4 mmol/L. We check if there is a difference in fasting glucose levels between the patients with bipolar disorder and the general population.

A report of statistical analysis using SPSS:

One-Sample Statistics

	N	Mean	Std. Deviation	Std. Error Mean
fastglu	25	5.6668	1.12149	.22430

One-Sample Test

	Test Value = 4					
					95% Confidence Interval of the Difference	
	t	df	Sig. (2-tailed)	Mean Difference	Lower	Upper
fastglu	7.431	24	.000	1.66680	1.2039	2.1297

Report: There is significant difference in fasting glucose levels between bipolar patients and general population (M = 5.667; SD = 1.121; T = 7.431, df = 24, $p < 0.001$).

Independent T-test

The *independent T-test* is also called the *two-sample T-test.* It is a test used to determine if there is a statistically significant difference between the means of two unrelated groups. (See figure above.)

Example: Is there a significant difference in body mass index (BMI) between the patients and control subjects?

Group Statistics

	Disease	N	Mean	Std. Deviation	Std. Error Mean
BMI	Bipolar	25	29.53	2.748	.550
	Con	24	26.22	1.330	.271

Independent Samples Test

		Levene's Test for Equality of Variances		t-test for Equality of Means					95% Confidence Interval of the Difference	
		F	Sig.	t	df	Sig. (2-tailed)	Mean Difference	Std. Error Difference	Lower	Upper
BMI	Equal variances assumed	9.925	.003	5.327	47	.000	3.308	.621	2.059	4.557
	Equal variances not assumed			5.397	34.965	.000	3.308	.613	2.064	4.552

Report: An independent-samples T-test was conducted to compare the BMI between the patients (Bipolar) and controls (Con). The results showed that the BMI was significantly higher in the patients than in controls (29.53 ± 2.748 and 26.22 ± 1.330, $t_{(47)} = 5.327$, $p < 0.001$).

Paired T-Test

The *paired T-test* or *dependent T-test* compares the mean values from two related samples or two variables for the same subject. It tests a "before and after" scenario. (See figure above.)

Example: Is there a significant difference in body fat composition (%) prior to and after twelve weeks of exercise?

Paired Samples Statistics

		Mean	N	Std. Deviation	Std. Error Mean
Pair 1	body fat % baseline	31.957	30	5.5681	1.0166
	body fat % W12	30.847	30	6.0279	1.1005

Paired Samples Test

		Paired Differences					t	df	Sig. (2-tailed)
					95% Confidence Interval of the Difference				
		Mean	Std. Deviation	Std. Error Mean	Lower	Upper			
Pair 1	body fat % baseline - body fat % W12	1.1100	1.0940	.1997	.7015	1.5185	5.557	29	.000

Report: The body fat composition before and after twelve weeks of exercise was 31.957 ± 5.5681 and 30.847 ± 6.0279. The difference was significant between the prior to and after exercise, t = 5.557, df = 29, $p < 0.001$, 2 tailed.

Example:

Table. Demographic and clinical characteristics of patients and healthy controls

Variables	Patients (n = 76)	Controls (n = 76)	*t*	*p*
Age (y)	26.34 ± 8.16	26.95 ± 6.67	0.45	0.65
Education (y)	12.14 ± 3.33	12.74 ± 3.40	1.08	0.28
Duration of illness (d)	37.26 ± 52.43	-		
BMI kg/m2	22.14 ± 2.54	21.97 ± 2.38	0.44	0.66
Systolic BP (mm Hg)	109.34 ± 11.98	107.83 ± 9.77	0.85	0.4
Diastolic BP (mm Hg)	73.22 ± 7.99	73.16 ± 8.24	0.05	0.96
HDL-C (mmol/l)	1.32 ± 0.36	1.33 ± 0.46	0.08	0.94
TG (mmol/l)	1.24 ± 0.87	1.28 ± 0.65	0.33	0.74
FBG (mmol/l)	4.71 ± 0.67	4.68 ± 0.58	0.3	0.76
Urea (mmol/l)	4.56 ± 1.31	4.24 ± 0.96	1.76	0.08

Creatinine (μmol/l)	74.62 ± 18.61	70.04 ± 15.86	1.63	0.11
UA (μmol/l)	378.55 ± 99.08	293.39 ± 71.40	6.22	0.01

Abbreviations: BMI, body mass index; BP, blood pressure; HDL-C, high-density lipoprotein cholesterol; TG, triglyceride; FBG, fasting blood glucose levels; UA, uric acid. Data were extracted and modified from a paper (Chen et al., 2019).

Example: A scatter plot shows T-test results.

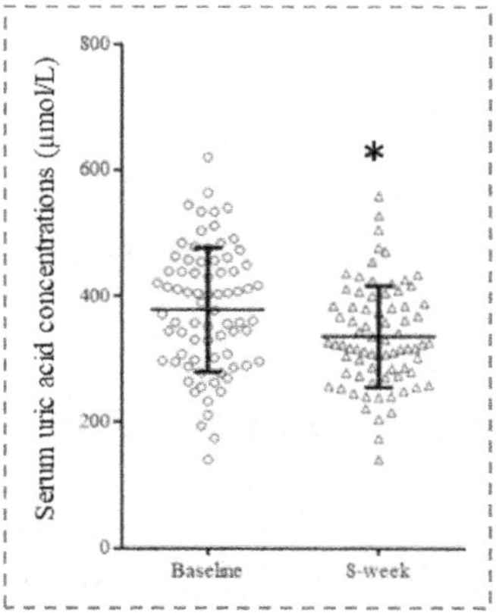

The figure shows the serum uric acid concentrations of bipolar disorder patients at baseline and eight weeks after the treatments. The figure was adapted and modified from our paper (Chen et al., 2019).

Pearson Correlation Coefficient

The *Pearson correlation coefficient test* is also called *Pearson's* r or the *bivariate correlation.* This analysis evaluates the linear correlation between two data sets and the relationship's strength.

A high association means that the variables have a strong relationship. It is noted that correlation is not necessarily causation.

Assumptions of a Pearson correlation coefficient are as follows:

- The data is distributed normally.
- There are similar variances between groups.
- Data are continuous.

Units

Two variables do not have to have the same units. For example, you may correlate a person's height (e.g., cm) with their body weight (e.g., kg).

Independent and Dependent Variables

This test does not respect variable types, regardless of the independent or dependent variable. For example, a researcher wants to study whether swimming speed performance correlates with a person's height. Let us say the *r* value is 0.61. The height increases, and so does swimming performance. When you plot another way, swimming to height also has an *r* value of 0.61. Therefore, this test does not respect the variables.

Pearson correlation allows us to report the following points:

- If the correlation is significant
- How strong the correlation is
- If it is a positive or negative correlation

Three Values in the Pearson Correlation

- r: Correlation coefficient
- r^2: Coefficient of determination
- k^2: Coefficient of non-determination

The Pearson correlation coefficient aims to understand the relationship between two quantitative and continuous variables.

Analysis and presentation: The correlation can be shown in a scatter plot of variables to verify linearity. Usually, the independent variable is on the x-axis and the dependent variable is on the y-axis.

Measurement: Range of correlation: –1.0 to 1.0.

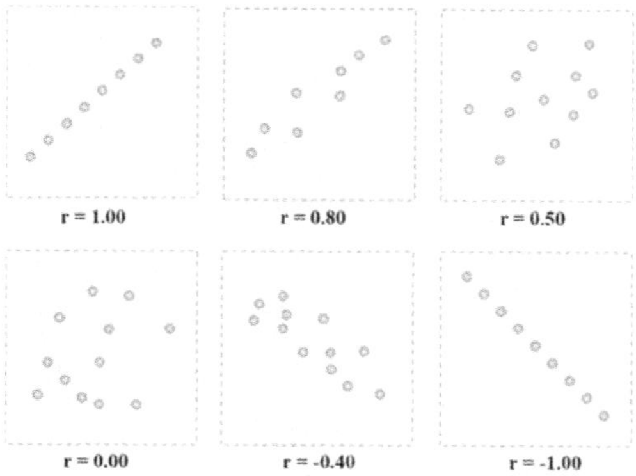

The figure depicts relationships between the two variables using a correlation coefficient. Correlation refers to the strength of a relationship. The above plots visually show their relationships.

R Value

The *r value* is a measure of the linear correlation between two variables.

- The *r* value ranges from +1 to -1.

- A total positive linear correlation is +1.
- No linear correlation is 0.
- A total negative linear correlation is -1.

The Strength of the Correlation

- 0.25 is a weak correlation.
- 0.26 to 0.50 is a moderate correlation.
- 0.51 to 0.75 is a fair correlation.
- 0.76 to 1 is a strong correlation.

Example:

Researchers want to determine the correlation between body weight and waist size in a group of patients who have bipolar disorders.

Tests of Normality

	Kolmogorov-Smirnov[a]			Shapiro-Wilk		
	Statistic	df	Sig.	Statistic	df	Sig.
WC	.078	49	.200*	.984	49	.746
Weight1 Baseline	.103	49	.200*	.973	49	.311

*. This is a lower bound of the true significance.

a. Lilliefors Significance Correction

Report: A Shapiro-Wilk test shows that p = 0.746 in waist circumference and p = 0.311 in body weight. Both *p*-values are greater than 0.05. We accept the H_0 hypothesis. The test of normality shows that the data is distributed normally.

Correlations

		WC	Weight1Baseline
WC	Pearson Correlation	1	.636**
	Sig. (2-tailed)		.000
	N	49	49
Weight1Baseline	Pearson Correlation	.636**	1
	Sig. (2-tailed)	.000	
	N	49	49

**. Correlation is significant at the 0.01 level (2-tailed).

Report: A Pearson correlation analysis examines the relationship between an individual's weight and waist circumference. There was a significant positive correlation between weight and waist circumference ($r = 0.636$, $p < 0.001$, two-tailed, n = 49).

Coefficient of Determination

The coefficient of determination ($\boldsymbol{r^2}$) allows more visualized representation, percentagewise.

Example: $r = 0.19$, $r^2 = 0.036$ or 3.6%

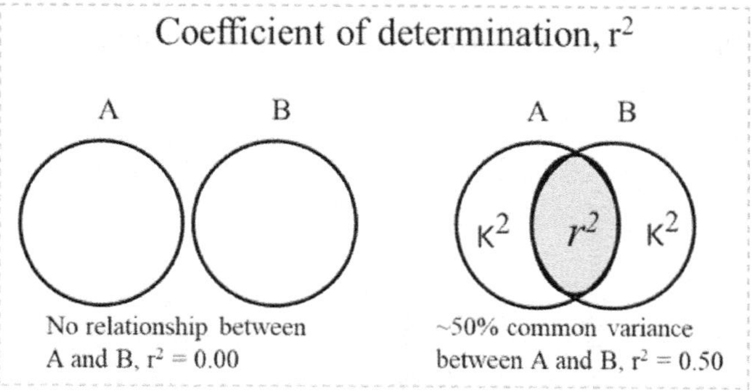

The figure above shows the coefficient of determination. An r^2 can be seen representing the correlated areas of two circles.

Coefficient of Non-Determination, K^2

- $K^2 = (1 - r^2)$ represents the proportion of variance NOT explained. *Example:* $r = 0.63$.
- The coefficient of determination is $r^2 = 0.397$; correlation 39.7%.
- The coefficient of non-determination is $K^2 = 0.603$, 60.3% (not correlated).

The coefficient of non-determination K^2 represents the non-correlated regions of the two circles.

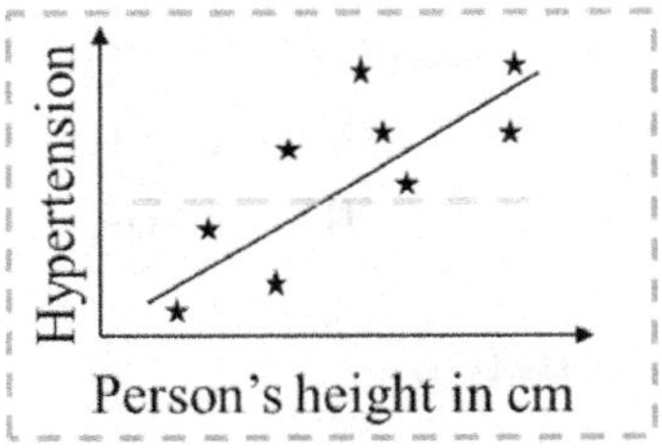

Non-sense correlation: The figure shows a positive correlation between the person's height and hypertension. Although statistical analysis shows significance, it does not make sense. Therefore, an interpretation needs to be cautious.

Example:

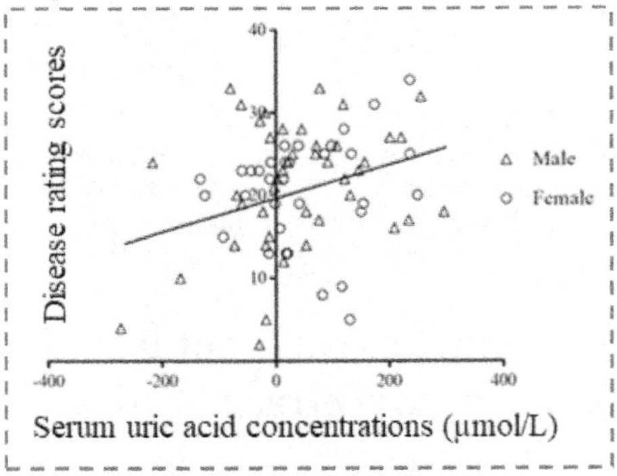

The above figure shows the correlation between serum uric acid concentrations and disease scores. The figure was adapted and modified from our paper (Chen et al., 2019).

Correlation Matrix

A correlation matrix is a summary of the data correlation. This type of plot shows the correlation coefficient (r) of multiple variables at a single time point. It reveals the strength and direction of relationships.

A correlation matrix plot is a good starting point before entering into a more advanced analysis to find potential *covariance.*

Assumptions of the Pearson correlation matrix are as follows:

Data is distributed normally.

Variability between groups is about equal.

Variables are in a linear relationship.

Besides the Pearson correlation matrix, you may use Spearman and Kendall rank-based correlation tests for nonparametric data analysis.

Example: Correlation coefficient matrix

Correlations

		education	Hcy	BDNFpgml	NRG1pgml
education	Pearson Correlation	1	-.113	.446**	-.168
	Sig. (2-tailed)		.287	.000	.118
	N	91	91	88	88
Hcy	Pearson Correlation	-.113	1	-.007	.030
	Sig. (2-tailed)	.287		.946	.780
	N	91	91	88	88
BDNFpgml	Pearson Correlation	.446**	-.007	1	-.198
	Sig. (2-tailed)	.000	.946		.064
	N	88	88	88	88
NRG1pgml	Pearson Correlation	-.168	.030	-.198	1
	Sig. (2-tailed)	.118	.780	.064	
	N	88	88	88	88

**. Correlation is significant at the 0.01 level (2-tailed).

The above table is a correlation coefficient (*r*) matrix report. The correlation matrix table shows that education is correlated with blood concentrations of BDNF in patients with schizophrenia ($r = 0.446$, $p = 0.000$). No other significant correlations were found in the table. Abbreviations: Hcy: Homocysteine is a common amino acid in the blood. We obtain homocysteine mostly from eating meat. High levels of homocysteine link to the early development of heart disease. BDNF: Brain-derived neurotrophic factor which stimulates nerve growth. Nrg1: Neuregulin 1 is altered in some patients who have schizophrenia.

Simple Linear Regression

Regression: The regression includes simple linear, multiple linear, and logistic regressions, which can predict the value of the outcome variables.

A simple linear regression aims to model the relationship between one independent variable and one dependent variable using a linear line, which is used to predict the event. Both variables are quantitative data. A simple linear regression establishes a model for an event prediction.

Assumptions of simple linear regression:

- Data are quantitative and have constant variance.
- The relationship between independent and dependent variables is linear.
- Data are normal distribution.

Example 1: Linear regression

You can use linear regression to study the following questions (r^2 and β values).

- A high-fat diet may increase body weight gain and weaken muscle strength and heart function. In this case, you can perform linear regression between the two continuous variables, body weight gain and muscle strength.
- Does more education lead me to earn more money?
- Does hot weather cause people to drink more water?
- Do heights predict body weight based on one hundred participants in a study?

Example 2: Here is a predictive question where you can generate a model.

Can bodyweight be used to predict waist size in a group of bipolar patients? Simple linear regression predicts waist size (dependent variable) based on body weight (independent variable) in a cohort of forty-nine bipolar patients.

Descriptive Statistics

	Mean	Std. Deviation	N
Waist Circumference	98.29	10.720	49
Weight	80.13	11.700	49

Report: A descriptive statistical analysis shows that the waist circumference was 98.29 ± 10.72 cm, and body weight was 80.13 ± 11.70 kg in forty-nine patients.

ANOVA[a]

Model		Sum of Squares	df	Mean Square	F	Sig.
1	Regression	2231.833	1	2231.833	31.940	.000[b]
	Residual	3284.167	47	69.876		
	Total	5516.000	48			

a. Dependent Variable: WaistCircumference_cm

b. Predictors: (Constant), Weight_Kg

Report: A SPSS ANOVA test shows that a significant regression equation was found F(1, 47) = 31.94, p < 0.001.

Model Summary[b]

					Change Statistics				
Model	R	R Square	Adjusted R Square	Std. Error of the Estimate	R Square Change	F Change	df1	df2	Sig. F Change
1	.636[a]	.405	.392	8.359	.405	31.940	1	47	.000

a. Predictors: (Constant), Weight

b. Dependent Variable: Waist Circumference

Report: Model summary shows that the r^2 is 0.405, $p < 0.001$.

Coefficients[a]

		Unstandardized Coefficients		Standardized Coefficients			Correlations		
Model		B	Std. Error	Beta	t	Sig.	Zero-order	Partial	Part
1	(Constant)	51.584	8.349		6.178	.000			
	Weight	.583	.103	.636	5.652	.000	.636	.636	.636

a. Dependent Variable: Waist Circumference

Report: Coefficients show that the participants' predicted waist size is 51.584 (β) + 0.583 cm when kilograms measure weight. This means that for every 1 kg increase in body weight of this population, the prediction is that there is a corresponding increase in waist size of 0.583 cm.

linear regression scatterplot

You can use fitted regression lines to determine the theoretical model, i.e., to illustrate the relationship between a predictor variable (independent) and a response variable (dependent).

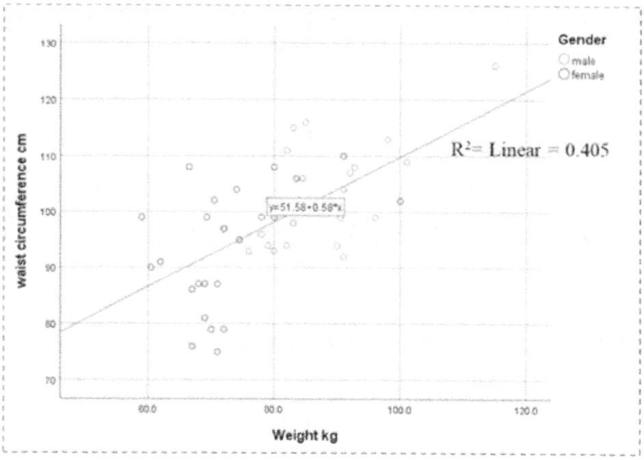

Report: The linear regression scatterplot shows the linear regression graph between body weight (kg) and waist circumferences (cm). R^2 linear = 0.405, y = 51.58 + 0.58*x

Multiple Linear Regression

The difference between simple linear regression and multiple linear regression is the number of independent variables (IVs) (See figure below.) Multiple linear regression uses multiple independent variables on one dependent variable, e.g., the effect of age, years of education, diabetes, and gender (IV) on memory (DV).

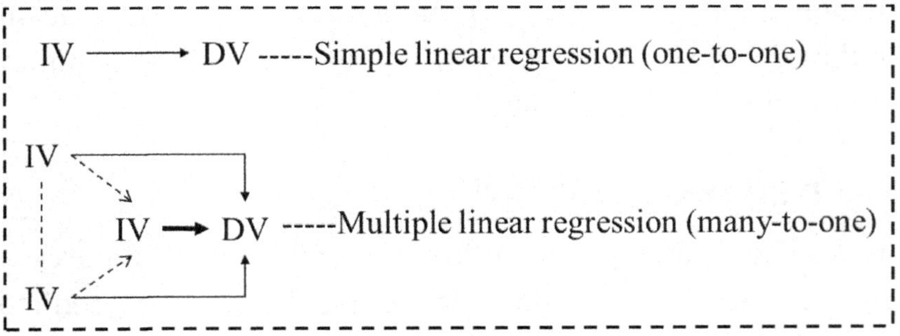

The Question Requires a Multiple Regression Analysis

Example:

Can work experience and schooling predict earning? Here, the first independent variable is work experience, the second independent variable is schooling, and the dependent variable is earnings.

It is noted that both simple and multiple linear regressions do *not* give the causal effect.

Binary Logistic Regression

A *binary logistic regression* is a regression analysis that the outcome variable is binary. The dependent variable is binary, or there are only two outcomes. *Examples:* Binary variables are black or red, death or no death, recovery or no recovery, and obesity or no obesity.

An example question:

Is there a probability of heavy smokers developing lung cancer? This is either a yes or no question.

The assumptions of binary logistic regression are as follows:

- The dependent variable should be dichotomous, for example, presence and absence.
- The data should have no outliers.
- There should be no high correlations among the predictors, which a correlation matrix can assess among the predictors.

Example:

Researchers want to investigate whether or not there is a relationship between gender and color preference. Gender is male or female, and color preference is black or red. Gender is an independent variable. Color is a dependent variable.

The male group has 114 subjects, with 103 preferring black and 11 preferring red. The female group has 746 subjects, with 341 preferring black and 405 preferring red.

The odds ratio of preferring black for males vs. females is = (103/11)/(341/405) = 11.12. Therefore, a male has an eleven times higher chance of selecting a black than a female. The odds ratio of preferring red for male vs. female is = (11/103)/(405/341) = 0.09; 9%. Males have a 91% (1-0.09) lower odds of preferring red than females.

Note: You can use one or more independent variables (predictors) to *determine* an outcome variable.

Difference Between Linear Regression and Logistic Regression

Linear regression: The dependent variable is continuous.

Logistic regression: The dependent variable is binary or has only two outcomes. You can use one or more independent variables (predictors) to predict an outcome (either categorical or continuous). This is used to predict the odds.

Analysis of Variance

The analysis of variance (ANOVA) is a parametric test including one-way ANOVA, two-way ANOVA, and more. It examines statistical differences between the means of three or more groups. Usually, the T-test is used to analyze two group differences; however, you can also use ANOVA for two-group analysis.

Underlying assumptions of an ANOVA are as follows:

Independent variable:

- Independent groups are the treatment group(s) and control group.
- There is no relationship between the groups, e.g., participants should not be in more than one group.

Dependent variable:

- The data is distributed normally (examined by Shapiro-Wilk test).
- The data has homogeneity of variance (examined by Levene's test).
- It requires continuous data.
- It requires an absence of outliers.

One-Way ANOVA

A one-way ANOVA is known as a one-factor ANOVA and parametric test. One-way ANOVA determines possible differences between three or more means. The difference between one-way and two-way ANOVAs is the number of independent variables. The one-way ANOVA has one independent variable (one factor); however, the two-way ANOVA has two independent (two factors) variables.

There is a two-step process:

- Step 1. It is to detect if there is an overall difference among the groups. But this does not tell where the difference lies.
- Step 2. After the ANOVA shows a statistical significance, you can perform post hoc analysis. A post hoc analysis allows the identification of where the differences lie.

The independent variable can have several levels, such as low, medium, and high doses of an anti-diabetic drug, or an intervention in different groups (young and old) of participants.

Example:

Psychiatrists want to investigate if the mean body weights differ among male bipolar, male normal, female bipolar, and female normal subjects.

Descriptives

weight

					95% Confidence Interval for Mean			
	N	Mean	Std. Deviation	Std. Error	Lower Bound	Upper Bound	Minimum	Maximum
MaleBipolar	13	92.592	8.5461	2.3703	87.428	97.757	83.0	115.0
MaleControl	12	76.958	11.3006	3.2622	69.778	84.138	60.5	100.0
FemaleBipolar	12	81.500	5.6969	1.6446	77.880	85.120	72.0	92.0
FemaleNormal	12	68.442	3.4490	.9956	66.250	70.633	59.0	72.0
Total	49	80.133	11.7000	1.6714	76.772	83.493	59.0	115.0

Report: Descriptive statistics report the mean and standard deviation values. A descriptive analysis shows that the mean values of body weight were 92.59 ± 8.55 kg in the bipolar male group (n = 13); 76.96 ± 11.30 kg in the male control group (n = 12); 81.50 ± 5.70 kg in the bipolar female group (n =12); and 68.44 ± 3.45 kg in the female control group (n = 12). The report also gives the lower and upper bound values in 95% confidence intervals of the mean.

ANOVA

weight

	Sum of Squares	df	Mean Square	F	Sig.
Between Groups	3801.660	3	1267.220	20.594	.000
Within Groups	2769.008	45	61.534		
Total	6570.668	48			

Report: The one-way ANOVA shows a significant difference in body weight among the four groups, $F_{(3, 45)} = 20.59$, $p < 0.001$. Since the *p*-value is less than 0.05, multiple post hoc comparisons should be performed to determine where the differences lie.

Multiple Comparisons

Dependent Variable: weight
Tukey HSD

(I) Subgroups	(J) Subgroups	Mean Difference (I-J)	Std. Error	Sig.	95% Confidence Interval Lower Bound	Upper Bound
MaleBipolar	MaleControl	15.6340*	3.1402	.000	7.257	24.011
	FemaleBipolar	11.0923*	3.1402	.005	2.715	19.470
	FemaleNormal	24.1506*	3.1402	.000	15.773	32.528
MaleControl	MaleBipolar	-15.6340*	3.1402	.000	-24.011	-7.257
	FemaleBipolar	-4.5417	3.2024	.495	-13.085	4.001
	FemaleNormal	8.5167	3.2024	.051	-.026	17.060
FemaleBipolar	MaleBipolar	-11.0923*	3.1402	.005	-19.470	-2.715
	MaleControl	4.5417	3.2024	.495	-4.001	13.085
	FemaleNormal	13.0583*	3.2024	.001	4.515	21.601
FemaleNormal	MaleBipolar	-24.1506*	3.1402	.000	-32.528	-15.773
	MaleControl	-8.5167	3.2024	.051	-17.060	.026
	FemaleBipolar	-13.0583*	3.2024	.001	-21.601	-4.515

*. The mean difference is significant at the 0.05 level.

Report: Multiple comparisons are Tukey's HSD (honestly significant difference) analyses: indicates that the mean difference is significant at $p < 0.05$. The bipolar male group had a significantly heavier body weight than the healthy male control group ($p = 0.000$). Similarly, the female bipolar group had a significantly heavier body weight than the female control group ($p = 0.001$).

Post Hoc Analysis

A post hoc analysis determines where the differences truly come from after an ANOVA shows significant results ($p<0.05$).

Which Post Hoc Test to Use

Although there are many post hoc tests, most give similar results; however, the test you choose can make a difference if the effect size is small. It also depends on the research questions if you chase minor changes.

You should choose a conservative analysis if it has important implications (life and death). In this case, choosing the most generous post hoc analysis is not appropriate. On the other hand, missing an actual difference is possible when you use the most conservative analysis. For example, if the sample size is small, you could penalize yourself by choosing a conservative test.

Choices of Post Hoc Tests

If a *p*-value of the ANOVA is less than 0.05, it requires a post hoc analysis.

The procedure is (1) to check if there is an equal variance (Levene's test). If the data do not have equal variance, you can use the Games-Howell test. If the data have equal variance, you may check if there is an equal sample size (or end). (2). If the data have an equal or similar sample size, you can use Tukey's HDS or REGWQ. (3) If the data slightly differs in sample size (e.g., n = 100 vs. n = 95), you can use the Gabriel test. If the data has a large difference in sample size (e.g., n = 100 vs. n = 70), you should use Hochbergi's GT2 test.

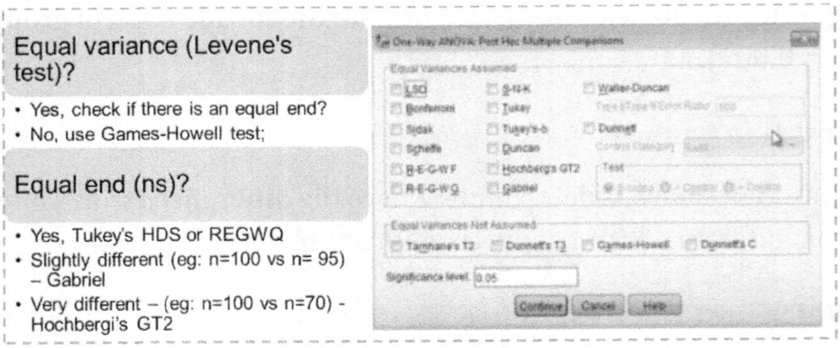

Bonferroni test: This test is conservative and stringent and controls for type I errors. However, it is less potent in detecting statistical significance.

Dunnett's test: This test compares the control condition against all other conditions. It does not compare experimental conditions to each other.

Example:

How to report the post hoc analysis? First, researchers want to know if there is a significant difference in body weight among the four subgroups of subjects, including male bipolar, male normal, female bipolar, and female normal subjects.

Post hoc comparisons between subgroups were made using Tukey's HSD test. Bonferroni corrections are applied to each test to adjust for multiple testing if the variables are from the same subjects.

One-Way Repeated Measures ANOVA

A repeated-measures ANOVA is a within-subjects ANOVA. It compares the means when the same subjects are measured more than twice; therefore, these means are related. For example, you measure the participants over multiple time points in response to an intervention, or you compare the reactions of the same participants to several trials.

"One-way" means that there is one factor in the experiment. It is the equivalent of the T-test or one-way ANOVA but for related and repeated observations.

Pretest and posttest: The same subjects are tested on several occasions, for example, pre-treatment, treatment, and post-treatment. This will be a within-subject ANOVA.

Example:

Researchers investigate the IQ scores of a group of participants at the baseline and at one and two months of training. In this example, IQ score is a dependent variable, whilst the independent variable is time. So here we have three readings: baseline, one, and two months of training.

- Pretest and Posttest design
  - Within-subject design having more than two measures
  - One independent variable or one treatment
- Example:
  - Intervention: Baseline - treatment - posttest 1 - posttest 2

Several independent variables for one dependent variable in the same participants: The same participants are measured on several independent variables.

Example:

Researchers want to investigate the taste preference of the same participants by having them each chocolate-, caramel-, and lemon-flavored foods. In this example, taste preference is your dependent variable, whilst the independent variable is the "conditions" which relate to the same participants.

- Several independent variables for one dependent variable in the same participants
  - Within-subject having more than two conditions
  - One dependent variable

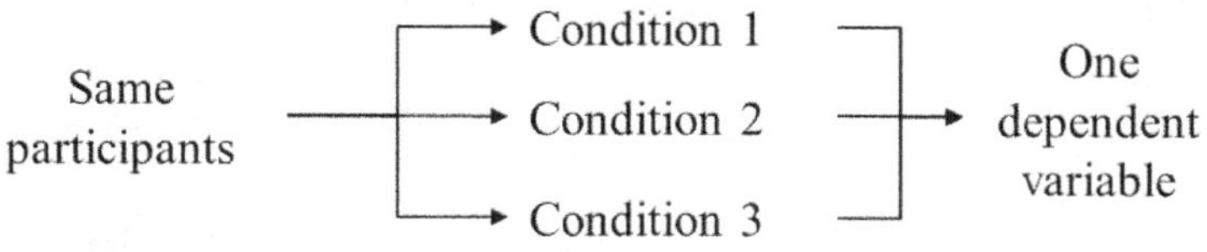

Several outcome variables for one independent variable in the same participants: Researchers can measure several outcome variables or dependent variables in the same participants having one independent variable.

- Several outcome variables for one independent variable in the same participants
  - Within-subject having one independent variable
  - Several outcome variables

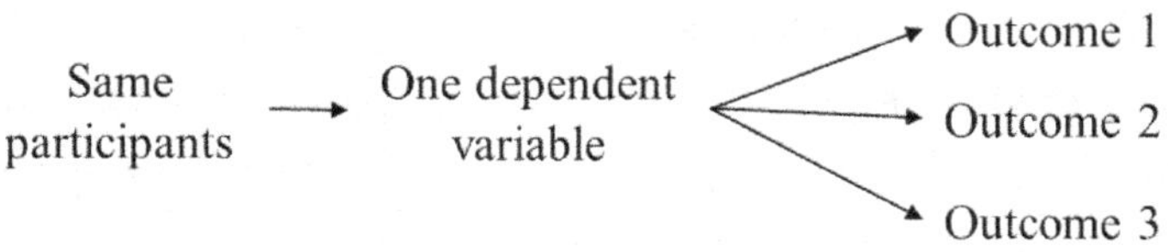

Example:

Researchers want to measure the chemical changes of ten brain structures in response to a high-fat diet, potentially regulating body weight in the same participants. Here, the independent variable is a high-fat diet. The dependent variables are the chemical changes of ten brain structures.

Advantages

This analysis controls individual differences and reduces variations because the same subjects are measured.

The study is economical because fewer subjects are required using repeated measures on the same participants.

Example:

The below example describes that researchers investigate whether there is a fat composition change after six and twelve weeks of exercise.

Tests of Within-Subjects Effects

Measure: MEASURE_1

Source		Type III Sum of Squares	df	Mean Square	F	Sig.
time	Sphericity Assumed	12.606	2	6.303	19.282	.000
	Greenhouse-Geisser	12.606	1.899	6.638	19.282	.000
	Huynh-Feldt	12.606	2.000	6.303	19.282	.000
	Lower-bound	12.606	1.000	12.606	19.282	.000
Error(time)	Sphericity Assumed	11.114	34	.327		
	Greenhouse-Geisser	11.114	32.286	.344		
	Huynh-Feldt	11.114	34.000	.327		
	Lower-bound	11.114	17.000	.654		

Report: A one-way repeated measures ANOVA with within-subjects tests showed that there was a significant effect among three time points measured, baseline and six and twelve weeks after exercise ($F(2, 34) = 19.283$, $p < 0.001$).

Pairwise Comparisons

Measure: MEASURE_1

(I) time	(J) time	Mean Difference (I-J)	Std. Error	Sig.[b]	95% Confidence Interval for Difference[b]	
					Lower Bound	Upper Bound
1	2	.833*	.192	.001	.324	1.343
	3	1.144*	.208	.000	.592	1.697
2	1	-.833*	.192	.001	-1.343	-.324
	3	.311	.170	.253	-.140	.762
3	1	-1.144*	.208	.000	-1.697	-.592
	2	-.311	.170	.253	-.762	.140

Based on estimated marginal means

*. The mean difference is significant at the .05 level.

b. Adjustment for multiple comparisons: Bonferroni.

Report: Pairwise comparisons showed that exercise reduced body fat percentage at week six ($p = 0.001$, group 2 vs. group 1) and week twelve ($p < 0.001$, group 3 vs. group 1) compared with baseline. Abbreviations: Sig^b: the adjustment for multiple comparisons with Bonferroni correction; 1: baseline; 2: six weeks of exercise; and 3: twelve weeks of exercise.

Two-Way ANOVA

A two-way ANOVA is a factorial analysis. It aims to compare two different categorical independent variables to one continuous dependent variable. It assesses the means of two categorical independent variables in combination to determine how they affect a dependent variable.

This type of analysis investigates if there is an *interaction* between the two categorical independent variables on the dependent variable. The interaction occurs when one independent variable affects the outcome variable depending on another variable. For example, anxiety may be affected by physical activity depending on sex.

If there is a significant interaction between the independent variables, further analysis is required to determine where the main impact lies.

Example:

A researcher wants to know whether or not there is a difference in waist size between the patients and controls and sex differences. It requires a typical factorial design with two independent factors and two levels, comparing bipolar males, control males, bipolar females, and control females. Therefore, researchers use a two-way ANOVA for four-group analysis.

Descriptive Statistics

Dependent Variable: WaistCircumference_cm

Gender	Disease	Mean	Std. Deviation	N
male	Bipolar	106.08	9.716	13
	Con	99.25	5.926	12
	Total	102.80	8.684	25
female	Bipolar	99.00	7.348	12
	Con	88.17	11.150	12
	Total	93.58	10.766	24
Total	Bipolar	102.68	9.218	25
	Con	93.71	10.407	24
	Total	98.29	10.720	49

Report: A two-way ANOVA has descriptive statistics showing the mean values and their respective standard deviations and also sample sizes (n)

Tests of Between-Subjects Effects

Dependent Variable: WaistCircumference_cm

Source	Type III Sum of Squares	df	Mean Square	F	Sig.	Partial Eta Squared
Corrected Model	2035.160[a]	3	678.387	8.770	.000	.369
Intercept	471215.490	1	471215.490	6091.834	.000	.993
Gender	1008.784	1	1008.784	13.041	.001	.225
Disease	954.000	1	954.000	12.333	.001	.215
Gender * Disease	49.098	1	49.098	.635	.430	.014
Error	3480.840	45	77.352			
Total	478860.000	49				
Corrected Total	5516.000	48				

a. R Squared = .369 (Adjusted R Squared = .327)

Report: A two-way ANOVA was performed to examine the effect of gender and disease on waist circumference values. The two-way ANOVA revealed there was a significant effect of gender ($F_{(1, 45)}$ = 13.041, p = 0.001) and disease ($F_{(1,45)}$ = 12.333, p = 0.001), however no interaction of gender and disease ($F_{(1,45)}$ = 0.635, p = 0.430).

A Two-Way ANOVA versus a One-Way ANOVA Design

	Two-way ANOVA				One-way ANOVA				
	Two categories				One category				
	four group design				two group design		three group design		
	G1	G2	G3	G4	G1	G2	G1	G2	G3
IV-1*	-	-	+	+	+	+	-	+	+
IV-2*	-	+	-	+	-	+	-	-	+
	This design can examine the interaction between 2 independent variables.				Here are two designs. Both cannot address the interaction between two independent variables.				

*: IV-1 and IV-2 are independent variables one and two.

Note: If you want to examine the *interactions* between two categorical independent variables, you use a two-way ANOVA. The design will require each independent variable group to have two levels. Therefore, it will be four groups. However, a one-way ANOVA does not address the interaction and can be two or three groups.

Two-Way Repeated-Measures ANOVA

A *two-way repeated-measure ANOVA* is also called a *two-factor repeated-measures ANOVA*. *Two factors* refers to two categorical variables, for example, different treatments and different conditions. Repeated measures mean that the dependent variables are measured more than once, or an extension of a paired T-test is used to compare the means over multiple time points.

It evaluates the effect of two within-subject unrelated independent variables on a dependent variable. The purpose is to examine if there is a statistically significant interaction effect between two within-subjects independent variables on a dependent variable.

It is a mix of between- and within-subjects design and requires repeated-measure ANOVA.

It investigates the dependent variables of two or more groups (factors) over two or more time points.

Example: Two-Way Repeated-Measures ANOVA

Researchers hypothesized that the bodyweight changes are different between the swimming and running exercise protocols measured every six weeks for up to twenty-four weeks.

	Bodyweight (Kg, Weeks)				
	0	6	12	18	24
Swimming					
Running					

The study will be a two-group pretest-posttest design because two categorical independent variables (swimming and running) require a two-way ANOVA. In addition, the body weight changes are measured in the same subjects multiple times, requiring a repeated measure ANOVA. Therefore, it requires a mix of between-group and within-group design.

The two groups are a swimming group and a running group. You may ask if there is an interaction between two different exercise protocols for body weight changes over a period. The statistical analysis should be a two-way repeated-measures ANOVA.

Analysis of Covariance

An *analysis of covariance*, ANCOVA, examines the differences in the mean values of a dependent variable whilst controlling for independent variables that are not of primary interest (covariates). The ANCOVA aims to remove covariates and then calculate based on the remaining dependent variables.

This analysis has at least one categorical independent variable (factor) and another independent variable (covariate).

Baseline data: The ANCOVA is used when performing pretest and posttest analyses because posttest variables may be affected by a pretest covariate. An ANCOVA can remove the confounding factors when there are baseline differences between the intervention and control groups. Some common confounding factors are age, education, etc.

Association matrix: An *association matrix analysis* can be used as the first step to search for possible covariates.

Non-related concept: This analysis is useful when the confounding factor is linearly related to the outcome but not conceptually related to the factors.

Adjusted mean: ANCOVA reports the differences of adjusted means (i.e., adjusted for covariate).

Recommended Steps for ANCOVA:

1) Perform an association matrix analysis to search for possible covariates.
2) Find significant associations.
3) Perform an ANCOVA on those variables.

Underlying Assumptions of a One-Way ANCOVA

- The independent variable consists of two or more categorical independent groups.
- The dependent variables should be on a continuous scale.
- There should be no significant outliers.
- The residuals should be approximately normally distributed for each variable.
- There needs to be homogeneity of variances.

Example:

Researchers want to investigate whether or not there is a difference in waist circumference between male and female patients who have bipolar disorder. The doctor suspects that smoking may affect waist size. Therefore, a research design uses an ANCOVA controlling for smoking.

Descriptive Statistics

Dependent Variable: WaistCircumference_cm

Gender	Mean	Std. Deviation	N
male	102.80	8.684	25
female	93.58	10.766	24
Total	98.29	10.720	49

Report: Descriptive statistics show that waist sizes are 102.80 ± 8.684 cm in males (n = 25) and 93.58 ± 10.766 in females (n = 24).

Tests of Between-Subjects Effects

Dependent Variable: WaistCircumference_cm

Source	Type III Sum of Squares	df	Mean Square	F	Sig.
Corrected Model	1682.764[a]	2	841.382	10.097	.000
Intercept	70517.465	1	70517.465	846.231	.000
Smoking	642.597	1	642.597	7.711	.008
Gender	353.533	1	353.533	4.243	.045
Error	3833.236	46	83.331		
Total	478860.000	49			
Corrected Total	5516.000	48			

a. R Squared = .305 (Adjusted R Squared = .275)

Report: After adjusting scores for smoking, there was still a significant difference between the males and females in waist size F(1, 46) = 7.711, p = 0.008]. Therefore, gender had significant effects in waist size, F(1, 46) = 4.243, p = 0.045.

Estimates

Dependent Variable: WaistCircumference_cm

Gender	Mean	Std. Error	95% Confidence Interval Lower Bound	Upper Bound
male	101.179[a]	1.917	97.321	105.037
female	95.272[a]	1.960	91.326	99.217

a. Covariates appearing in the model are evaluated at the following values: Smoking = .80.

Adjusted means

Report: The adjusted values were 101.179 ± 1.917 cm in males and 95.272 ± 1.960 cm in females. These numbers were slightly different from the pre-adjustment values.

The Table Depicts Similarities and Differences between ANOVA and ANCOVA

ANOVA	ANCOVA
Examines the differences between two or more independent variables on a dependent variable. Examines the differences between group means.	Is an extension of the ANOVA but incorporates a covariate. Uses adjusted means or adjusted for the covariate. Is a statistic control for a third variable, confounding variable, or covariate, which could affect the results.

ASK YOURSELF
▪ What is the aim of a T-test? ▪ What are the underlying assumptions of a T-test? ▪ When do you need to use a one-sample T-test? ▪ When do you need to use an independent T-test? ▪ When do you need to use a paired T-test? ▪ What will a Pearson correlation coefficient test tell you? ▪ What do r, r^2 and k^2 mean? ▪ What type of research question requires a correlation matrix analysis to answer it? ▪ What are the similarities and differences between simple linear regression, multiple linear regression, and logistic regression? ▪ When should you use a one-way ANOVA? ▪ When should you perform a post hoc analysis? How do you select an appropriate type of post hoc analysis? ▪ What type of data requires a one-way repeated-measures ANOVA? ▪ What does a two-way ANOVA test assess? ▪ When should you use a two-way repeated-measure ANOVA? ▪ When should you use an ANCOVA?

CHAPTER 10

Nonparametric Test

TOPIC OUTLINE

- Chi-square test
- Spearman's rank correlation coefficient
- Wilcoxon signed-rank test
- Mann-Whitney U test
- Kruskal-Wallis H test
- Friedman's ANOVA

The data used in nonparametric tests do not require to fit any normality or is a distribution-free test. The data may be collected from a sample that does not follow a specific distribution to represent that population.

Nonparametric tests are more general than parametric tests, as they are based on fewer assumptions about the data distribution; therefore, they are less potent than parametric analyses.

When Should You Consider Nonparametric Analysis?

Data distribution: Data does not require a normal distribution. When data is severely skewed, the study uses the medium to represent it.

Data variation: Data does not require homogeneity of variance between groups.

Data type: Data is nominal, ordinal, or ranking.

Outliers: The data has outliers, which cannot be removed.

Nonparametric tests include Spearman's rank correlation coefficient, Wilcoxon signed-rank test, Mann-Whitney U, Kruskal-Wallis H test, Friedman's ANOVA, and chi-square test.

Table: Measurements of Parametric and Nonparametric Analyses

	Parametric	Non-parametric
Dependent variable	Interval or ratio	Nominal, Ordinal, Interval, Ratio
Central measure	Mean	Median
Distribution	Normal	Any
Variance	Equal	Not equal

Equivalence of parametric and nonparametric analyses: Once the different parametric tests and their applications are understood, you can apply nonparametric analysis easily. For example, the Pearson test cannot determine correlation if the data is not in a normal distribution. So instead, use the nonparametric equivalent, the Spearman test.

Equivalence of parametric and nonparametric tests

Parametric analysis	Nonparametric analysis
Pearson *r*	Spearman *r* (rho) r_s
Paired T-test	Wilcoxon signed-rank test
Independent T-test	Mann-Whitney U test
One-way ANOVA	The Kruskall-Wallis test
One-way repeated measure	Friedman's ANOVA

Data that requires nonparametric analysis

Nominal data: E.g., blue, red, yellow.

Ordinal data: It includes ranking or order of sorts. Ordinal data consists of numerical scores, e.g., primary school, high school and university; none, mild, moderate, and severe; very satisfied, satisfied, OK, and dissatisfied.

Interval data: The interval data does not have a normal distribution or have unequal group variance.

Ratio data: The ratio data does not have a normal distribution or have unequal group variance.

Limitations or Potential Pitfalls of a Nonparametric Test

Nonparametric tests are usually *less powerful* than corresponding parametric tests; therefore, it is less likely to reject the null hypothesis when it is false, increasing the chance of a type II error.

Nonparametric tests often require the researcher to modify the hypotheses. For example, most nonparametric tests performed to investigate the population center value are about the *median* rather than the mean. However, if you have planned to investigate the mean value, you may use the median if the data is nonparametric.

Chi-Square Test

A chi-square or Pearson's chi-square (χ^2) test is a nonparametric test for categorical data, e.g., nominal or ordinal groups. It examines whether (1) the frequency distribution of a categorical variable is *different* between groups and (2) the association between two categorical variables.

Difference between Groups in One Categorical Variable

This allows you to test whether the frequency distribution of the categorical variable is significantly different from your expectations. Often, but not always, the expectation is that the categories will have equal proportions.

Example 1:

	Patients (n = 318)	Controls (n = 160)	χ^2 (df, n)	p
Male, n (%)	150 (47)	74 (46)	0.006	0.807
Smoker, n (%)	86 (27)	26 (16)	6.913	0.009
Married, n (%)	175 (55)	108 (68)	6.852	0.009
Overweight, n (%)	145 (46)	48 (30)	10.757	0.001
Hypertension, n (%)	91 (29)	29 (18)	6.231	0.013
MetS, n (%)	135 (43)	35 (22)	19.669	0.000

H_0 hypothesis: The patients and controls are smokers in equal proportions. *H_A hypothesis:* The patients and controls are smokers in different proportions. Data were extracted and modified from a paper (Chen et al., 2018).

Association in Two Categorical Variables:

The chi-square test allows you to test whether the two categorical variables are related.

Example 2:

Researchers want to investigate whether patients with bipolar disorder are associated with a high risk of smoking or are more likely to smoke. There were twenty-five patients and twenty-four healthy controls involved in this study. Here, the independent variables are disease and smoking. The research question is if they are related.

Disease * smoking Crosstabulation

Count

		smoking		
		not smoking	smoking	Total
Disease	Bipolar	0	25	25
	Con	10	14	24
Total		10	39	49

Report: The analysis shows that all bipolar patients are smokers, and control subjects have fourteen smokers and ten non-smokers.

Chi-Square Tests

	Value	df	Asymptotic Significance (2-sided)	Exact Sig. (2-sided)	Exact Sig. (1-sided)
Pearson Chi-Square	13.088[a]	1	.000		
Continuity Correction[b]	10.648	1	.001		
Likelihood Ratio	16.988	1	.000		
Fisher's Exact Test				.000	.000
Linear-by-Linear Association	12.821	1	.000		
N of Valid Cases	49				

a. 1 cells (25.0%) have expected count less than 5. The minimum expected count is 4.90.

b. Computed only for a 2x2 table

Report: Chi-square tests show a strong correlation between smoking and bipolar disorder: χ^2 (1, n = 49) = 13.088, p = 0.000. All bipolar patients were smokers in this case, and 58% of healthy subjects were smokers.

Example 3:

The chi-square test determines the association between the symptom and risk factors.

Table
Factors associated with metabolic syndrome and hyperuricemia

Variables	Hyperuricemia Yes (n = 86)	No (n = 232)	χ^2	*p*
MetS, n (%)	55 (62.5)	80 (34.8)	20.015	< 0.001
Increased WC, n (%)	63 (71.6)	123 (53.5)	8.600	0.003
Low HDL-C, n (%)	47 (53.4)	104 (45.2)	1.713	0.191
HTG, n (%)	44 (50.0)	74 (32.2)	8.666	0.003
Hypertension, n (%)	30 (34.1)	61 (26.5)	1.785	0.182
Hyperglycemia, n (%)	29 (33.0)	46 (20.0)	5.927	0.015

Abbreviations: MetS: metabolic syndrome, WC: waist circumference, HDL-C: high-density lipoprotein cholesterol, HTG, hypertriglyceridemia. MetS: has at least three of the following five components: (1) WC > 90 cm in men or 80 cm in women; (2) hypertriglyceridemia, triglycerides > 1.70 mmol/L (150 mg/dL); (3) high-density lipoprotein cholesterol (HDL-C), < 1.03 mmol/L (40 mg/dL) in men or 1.29 mmol/L (50 mg/dL) in women; (4) hypertension: blood pressure > 130 mmHg systolic or > 85 mmHg diastolic; and (5) hyperglycemia: fasting glucose concentration > 5.6 mmol/L (100 mg/dL). Hyperuricemia, serum uric acid > 420 µmol/L (7.0mg/dL) for men and > 360 µmol/L (6.0mg/dL) for women.

Report: The patients with hyperuricemia compared with patients without hyperuricemia had a higher prevalence of metabolic syndrome. Hyperuricemia was associated with increased waist circumference, hypertriglyceridemia, and hyperglycemia, but not with hypertension and low HDL-C in the patients. The table was adapted and modified from our previous paper (Chen et al., 2018).

Spearman's Rank Correlation Coefficient

A *Spearman's rank correlation coefficient test,* also called *Spearman's* r *test,* is the nonparametric version of the Pearson correlation, which tests the strength and direction of associations.

Rank: Spearman's *r* test is a nonparametric measure of rank correlation. It is related to statistical dependence between the ranking of two variables.

This is a nonparametric measure of association between two ranked (ordinal data) or other nonparametric variables.

Example 1:

Is there an association between blood triglyceride concentrations and young, middle-aged, and old patients (age rank)?

Correlations

			AgeRank	triglyceride
Spearman's rho	AgeRank	Correlation Coefficient	1.000	.259
		Sig. (2-tailed)	.	.072
		N	49	49
	triglyceride	Correlation Coefficient	.259	1.000
		Sig. (2-tailed)	.072	.
		N	49	49

Report: Spearman's rho analysis shows no significant correlation between the triglyceride levels and ranked age groups (r_s = 0.259, p = 0.072, two-tailed, n = 49).

Example 2:

A project manager recruits a doctor to join the team to diagnose the patients' diseases. The manager wants to determine if the newly recruited doctor can perform the same diagnosis for the same patients as the other team doctors. So the manager recruits eight patients. The diagnostic criteria are the scores in ranks, say from one to eight. The results show that the ranking scores between the newly recruited doctor and other doctors are highly correlated. Therefore, the recruited doctor is qualified to be a member of the research project.

Wilcoxon Signed-Rank Test

This test is the nonparametric equivalent of the *paired* samples T-test. It assesses if the ranked means differ when comparing two related samples, matched samples, or repeated measurements on the same subjects.

Example 1:

A researcher wants to investigate the differences between body fat percentages at baseline and twelve weeks after training in the same cohort of subjects. The data is nonparametric.

Descriptive Statistics

	N	Mean	Std. Deviation	Minimum	Maximum	Percentiles		
						25th	50th (Median)	75th
body fat % baseline	30	31.957	5.5681	19.5	44.9	28.000	30.900	35.600
body fat % W12	30	30.847	6.0279	17.3	44.8	25.625	30.600	34.475

Test Statistics[a]

	body fat % W12 - body fat % baseline
Z	-4.100[b]
Asymp. Sig. (2-tailed)	.000

a. Wilcoxon Signed Ranks Test

b. Based on positive ranks.

Report: The results showed a significant improvement in body fat percentage after twelve weeks of training. The median value was 30.9% at the baseline and 30.6% after twelve weeks of training. Z = -4.100, $p < 0.001$.

Mann-Whitney U

The *Mann-Whitney U test* compares differences between two independent groups when the dependent variable is either ordinal or nonparametric continuous data.

The Mann-Whitney U test is considered the nonparametric alternative to the independent T-test.

Example 1:

Are there any differences in the triglyceride levels (nonparametric data) between patients with bipolar disorder and healthy controls? There are two independent samples, equivalent to an independent T-test, but triglyceride data is nonparametric.

Statistics

triglyceride

Bipolar	N	Valid	25	Con	N	Valid	24
		Missing	0			Missing	0
	Mean		2.3736		Mean		1.1708
	Median		1.6100		Median		.9150
	Std. Deviation		1.51380		Std. Deviation		.64514
	Skewness		1.974		Skewness		.471
	Std. Error of Skewness		.464		Std. Error of Skewness		.472
	Kurtosis		3.449		Kurtosis		-1.201
	Std. Error of Kurtosis		.902		Std. Error of Kurtosis		.918
	Minimum		1.25		Minimum		.36
	Maximum		7.02		Maximum		2.34

Test Statistics[a]

	triglyceride
Mann-Whitney U	129.000
Wilcoxon W	429.000
Z	-3.421
Asymp. Sig. (2-tailed)	.001

a. Grouping Variable: Disease

Report: The Mann-Whitney analysis shows a significant difference in triglycerides between the patients and controls (U = 129, Z = -3.421, p = 0.001). The median value of triglycerides is 1.6100 for bipolar patients (n = 25) and 0.9150 for controls (n = 24).

Kruskal-Wallis H Test

The *Kruskal-Wallis H test* is the nonparametric equivalent of the one-way ANOVA and is also known as the one-way ANOVA on ranks.

The Kruskal-Wallis H test compares three or more groups of nonparametric data.

Example 1:

Researchers want to investigate if there are differences in triglyceride levels among male bipolar, male normal, female bipolar, and female normal. The data is nonparametric.

Test Statistics[a,b]

	triglyceride
Kruskal-Wallis H	14.367
df	3
Asymp. Sig.	.002

a. Kruskal Wallis Test

b. Grouping Variable: Subgroups

Report: The Kruskal-Wallis H report shows a significant difference in triglyceride among the four groups. Kruskal-Wallis H = 14.367, df = 3, p = 0.002.

Since there was a statistical difference, further tests were performed using a nonparametric test for each pair of independent sample comparisons. The Mann-Whitney U test will determine where the difference lies.

The descriptive statistical analysis provides the median values.

Friedman's ANOVA

Friedman's ANOVA is used for one-way repeated measures ANOVA by ranks. It is a nonparametric statistic test.

When should you use Friedman's ANOVA? When the same subjects are measured multiple times or the data is in ranks, ordinal, or nonparametric.

Example:

Researchers want to investigate the differences in body fat percentage at the baseline and after six and twelve weeks of training. (The data is nonparametric.)

Test Statistics[a]

N	30
Chi-Square	21.556
df	2
Asymp. Sig.	.000

a. Friedman Test

Report: The report shows a significant difference among the three groups analyzed by the Friedman test. Chi-square = 21.556, df = 2, p = 0.000.

Since there is a significant difference, a post hoc analysis is required to find where the difference lies. A post hoc analysis can be performed between baseline and week six, between baseline and week twelve and between weeks six and twelve.

Here, we need a Bonferroni correction to set the alpha value at 0.05/3 time points = 0.017. The significance level $p < 0.017$ will be used. You can use descriptive statistics to show the frequency of median values.

Ask yourself

- When should you consider nonparametric analysis?
- What are the differences between parametric and nonparametric analysis?
- What are the equivalent nonparametric versions of the parametric tests?
- What types of data require nonparametric analysis?
- What are the limitations or potential pitfalls of nonparametric testing?
- When should you use a Spearman's *r* test?
- When should you use Wilcoxon signed-rank test?
- What types of data require a Mann-Whitney U test?
- When should you use a Kruskal-Wallis test?
- When should you use Friedman's ANOVA test?
- What types of data require a chi-square test?

References

Akobeng, A.K., 2005. Principles of evidence based medicine. Arch Dis Child. 90, 837-40.

An, H., et al., 2018. Serum NCAM levels and cognitive deficits in first episode schizophrenia patients versus health controls. Schizophr Res. 192, 457-458.

Azevedo, A., Machado, A.P., Barros, H., 1999. Tobacco smoking among Portuguese high-school students. Bull World Health Organ. 77, 509-14.

Bastian, H., Glasziou, P., Chalmers, I., 2010. Seventy-five trials and eleven systematic reviews a day: how will we ever keep up? PLoS Med. 7, e1000326.

Chen, J., et al., 2018. Association between hyperuricemia and metabolic syndrome in patients suffering from bipolar disorder. BMC Psychiatry. 18, 390.

Chen, J.X., et al., 2019. Patients With Drug-Naive Bipolar Disorder in Remission After 8 Weeks of Treatment Had Decreased Serum Uric Acid Concentrations. Front Psychiatry. 10, 767.

Davies, G., et al., 2018. Long term extension of a randomised controlled trial of probiotics using electronic health records. Sci Rep. 8, 7668.

Dimitrov, D.M., Rumrill, P.D., Jr., 2003. Pretest-posttest designs and measurement of change. Work. 20, 159-65.

English, D.R., et al., 1998. Case-control study of sun exposure and squamous cell carcinoma of the skin. Int J Cancer. 77, 347-53.

Ghiasvand, R., et al., 2016. Sunscreen Use and Subsequent Melanoma Risk: A Population-Based Cohort Study. J Clin Oncol. 34, 3976-3983.

Gosho, M., Nagashima, K., Sato, Y., 2012. Study designs and statistical analyses for biomarker research. Sensors (Basel). 12, 8966-86.

Grodstein, F., et al., 1996. Postmenopausal estrogen and progestin use and the risk of cardiovascular disease. N Engl J Med. 335, 453-61.

Han, M., et al., 2013. Diabetes and cognitive deficits in chronic schizophrenia: a case-control study. PLoS One. 8, e66299.

Harris, A.D., et al., 2004. The use and interpretation of quasi-experimental studies in infectious diseases. Clin Infect Dis. 38, 1586-91.

Harris, A.D., et al., 2006. The use and interpretation of quasi-experimental studies in medical informatics. J Am Med Inform Assoc. 13, 16-23.

Huang, J., et al., 2022. The effects of probiotics plus dietary fiber on antipsychotic-induced weight gain: a randomized clinical trial. Transl Psychiatry. 12, 185.

Lipowicz, A., et al., 2015. Secular trends in BMI and the prevalence of obesity in young Polish males from 1965 to 2010. Eur J Public Health. 25, 279-82.

Llewellyn-Bennett, R., Bowman, L., Bulbulia, R., 2016. Post-trial follow-up methodology in large randomized controlled trials: a systematic review protocol. Syst Rev. 5, 214.

Mathes, T., Pieper, D., 2017. Clarifying the distinction between case series and cohort studies in systematic reviews of comparative studies: potential impact on body of evidence and workload. BMC Med Res Methodol. 17, 107.

McCambridge, J., Witton, J., Elbourne, D.R., 2014. Systematic review of the Hawthorne effect: new concepts are needed to study research participation effects. J Clin Epidemiol. 67, 267-77.

Nadkarni, P.S., Odejayi, G., 2014. Vitamin D and depression: A case series. SAGE Open Med Case Rep. 2, 2050313X14561570.

Nguyen, C., Suzuki, A., Bera, K., 2015. Use of Lorcaserin, A 5HT2C Agonist, In the Management of OlanzapineInduced Weight Gain. journal of Metabolic Syndrome. 4, 4-5.

Pan, F., et al., 2020. Factors associated with death outcome in patients with severe coronavirus disease-19 (COVID-19): a case-control study. Int J Med Sci. 17, 1281-1292.

Park, J.J.H., et al., 2021. Randomised trials at the level of the individual. Lancet Glob Health. 9, e691-e700.

Parnell, J.A., Reimer, R.A., 2009. Weight loss during oligofructose supplementation is associated with decreased ghrelin and increased peptide YY in overweight and obese adults. Am J Clin Nutr. 89, 1751-9.

Pennacchio, L.A., 2003. Insights from human/mouse genome comparisons. Mamm Genome. 14, 429-36.

Petersen, L.A., et al., 2000. Outcome of myocardial infarction in Veterans Health Administration patients as compared with medicare patients. N Engl J Med. 343, 1934-41.

Pourhoseingholi, M.A., Baghestani, A.R., Vahedi, M., 2012. How to control confounding effects by statistical analysis. Gastroenterol Hepatol Bed Bench. 5, 79-83.

Sackett, D.L., et al., 1996. Evidence based medicine: what it is and what it isn't. BMJ. 312, 71-2.

Sandroff, B.M., et al., 2018. Rationale and design of a single-blind, randomised controlled trial of exercise training for managing learning and memory impairment in persons with multiple sclerosis. BMJ Open. 8, e023231.

Straus, S.E., Sackett, D.L., 1998. Getting research findings into practice - Using research findings in clinical practice. British Medical Journal. 317, 339-342.

Suresh, K., 2011. An overview of randomization techniques: An unbiased assessment of outcome in clinical research. J Hum Reprod Sci. 4, 8-11.

Toots, A., et al., 2017. Effects of Exercise on Cognitive Function in Older People with Dementia: A Randomized Controlled Trial. J Alzheimers Dis. 60, 323-332.

Vickers, A.J., 2006. How to randomize. J Soc Integr Oncol. 4, 194-8.

Vintimilla, R., et al., 2019. The relationship of CRP and cognition in cognitively normal older Mexican Americans: A cross-sectional study of the HABLE cohort. Medicine (Baltimore). 98, e15605.

Wang, T.J., et al., 2013. 2-Aminoadipic acid is a biomarker for diabetes risk. J Clin Invest. 123, 4309-17.

Index

A

B

C

D

P

Q

R

S

T

U

W

Z

Made in the USA
Monee, IL
04 November 2026

67377571R00144